COVID-19 in Dentistry and Dental Education

COVID-19 in Dentistry and Dental Education

Editor

Giuseppe Alessandro Scardina

MDPI

Basel • Beijing • Wuhan • Barcelona • Belgrade • Novi Sad • Cluj • Manchester

Editor
Giuseppe Alessandro Scardina
Department of Surgical, Oncological
and Stomatological Disciplines,
Università degli Studi di Palermo
Palermo
Italy

Editorial Office
MDPI
St. Alban-Anlage 66
4052 Basel, Switzerland

This is a reprint of articles from the Special Issue published online in the open access journal *International Journal of Environmental Research and Public Health* (ISSN 1660-4601) (available at: https://www.mdpi.com/journal/ijerph/special_issues/covid_dentistry_dental_education).

For citation purposes, cite each article independently as indicated on the article page online and as indicated below:

Lastname, A.A.; Lastname, B.B. Article Title. *Journal Name* **Year**, *Volume Number*, Page Range.

ISBN 978-3-7258-0163-3 (Hbk)
ISBN 978-3-7258-0164-0 (PDF)
doi.org/10.3390/books978-3-7258-0164-0

Contents

Oana Tanculescu, Alina-Mihaela Apostu, Adrian Doloca, Sorina Mihaela Solomon, Diana Diaconu-Popa, Carmen Iulia Ciongradi, et al.
Perception of Remote Learning by Fixed Prosthodontic Students at a Romanian Faculty of Dentistry
Reprinted from: *Int. J. Environ. Res. Public Health* **2023**, *20*, 3622, doi:10.3390/ijerph20043622 . . . **1**

Katja Goetz, Hans-Jürgen Wenz and Katrin Hertrampf
Certainty in Uncertain Times: Dental Education during the COVID-19 Pandemic–A Qualitative Study
Reprinted from: *Int. J. Environ. Res. Public Health* **2023**, *20*, 3090, doi:10.3390/ijerph20043090 . . . **21**

Enzo Cumbo, Giuseppe Gallina, Pietro Messina and Giuseppe Alessandro Scardina
Filter Masks during the Second Phase of SARS-CoV-2: Study on Population
Reprinted from: *Int. J. Environ. Res. Public Health* **2023**, *20*, 2360, doi:10.3390/ijerph20032360 . . . **31**

Olesya V. Kytko, Yuriy L. Vasil'ev, Sergey S. Dydykin, Ekaterina Yu Diachkova, Maria V. Sankova, Tatiana M. Litvinova, et al.
COVID-19 Vaccinating Russian Medical Students—Challenges and Solutions: A Cross-Sectional Study
Reprinted from: *Int. J. Environ. Res. Public Health* **2022**, *19*, 11556, doi:10.3390/ijerph191811556 . **38**

Wasmiya Ali AlHayyan, Khalaf AlShammari, Falah AlAjmi and Sharat Chandra Pani
The Impact of COVID-19 on Dental Treatment in Kuwait—A Retrospective Analysis from the Nation's Largest Hospital
Reprinted from: *Int. J. Environ. Res. Public Health* **2022**, *19*, 9275, doi:10.3390/ijerph19159275 . . . **52**

Andrej Thurzo, Wanda Urbanová, Iveta Waczulíková, Veronika Kurilová, Bela Mriňáková, Helena Kosnáčová, et al.
Dental Care and Education Facing Highly Transmissible SARS-CoV-2 Variants: Prospective Biosafety Setting: Prospective, Single-Arm, Single-Center Study
Reprinted from: *Int. J. Environ. Res. Public Health* **2022**, *19*, 7693, doi:10.3390/ijerph19137693 . . . **60**

Azhar Iqbal, Kiran Kumar Ganji, Osama Khattak, Deepti Shrivastava, Kumar Chandan Srivastava, Bilal Arjumand, et al.
Enhancement of Skill Competencies in Operative Dentistry Using Procedure-Specific Educational Videos (E-Learning Tools) Post-COVID-19 Era—A Randomized Controlled Trial
Reprinted from: *Int. J. Environ. Res. Public Health* **2022**, *19*, 4135, doi:10.3390/ijerph19074135 . . . **85**

Deepak Nallaswamy Veeraiyan, Sheeja S. Varghese, Arvina Rajasekar, Mohmed Isaqali Karobari, Lakshmi Thangavelu, Anand Marya, et al.
Comparison of Interactive Teaching in Online and Offline Platforms among Dental Undergraduates
Reprinted from: *Int. J. Environ. Res. Public Health* **2022**, *19*, 3170, doi:10.3390/ijerph19063170 . . . **96**

Syed Nahid Basheer, Thilla Sekar Vinothkumar, Nassreen Hassan Mohammad Albar, Mohmed Isaqali Karobari, Apathsakayan Renugalakshmi, Ahmed Bokhari, et al.
Knowledge of COVID-19 Infection Guidelines among the Dental Health Care Professionals of Jazan Region, Saudi Arabia
Reprinted from: *Int. J. Environ. Res. Public Health* **2022**, *19*, 2034, doi:10.3390/ijerph19042034 . . . **104**

Matia Fazio, Christian Lombardo, Giuseppe Marino, Anand Marya, Pietro Messina, Giuseppe Alessandro Scardina, et al.
LinguAPP: An m-Health Application for Teledentistry Diagnostics
Reprinted from: *Int. J. Environ. Res. Public Health* **2022**, *19*, 822, doi:10.3390/ijerph19020822 . . . **117**

Ancuta Goriuc, Darius Sandu, Monica Tatarciuc and Ionut Luchian
The Impact of the COVID-19 Pandemic on Dentistry and Dental Education: A Narrative Review
Reprinted from: *Int. J. Environ. Res. Public Health* **2022**, *19*, 2537, doi:10.3390/ijerph19052537 . . . **129**

International Journal of
Environmental Research and Public Health

MDPI

Article

Perception of Remote Learning by Fixed Prosthodontic Students at a Romanian Faculty of Dentistry

Oana Tanculescu [1,†], Alina-Mihaela Apostu [1,*], Adrian Doloca [2,*], Sorina Mihaela Solomon [3,*], Diana Diaconu-Popa [4,†], Carmen Iulia Ciongradi [5,†], Raluca-Maria Vieriu [6,†], Ovidiu Aungurencei [1,†], Ana-Maria Fatu [7,†], Nicoleta Ioanid [1], Mihaela Scurtu [1,†] and Catalina Iulia Saveanu [8]

1 Discipline of Fixed Prosthodontics, Department of Odontology–Periodontology and Fixed Prosthodontics, Faculty of Dental Medicine, Grigore T. Popa University of Medicine and Pharmacy, 700115 Iasi, Romania
2 Discipline of Medical Informatics and Biostatistics, Department of Preventive Medicine and Interdisciplinarity, Faculty of Dental Medicine, Grigore T. Popa University of Medicine and Pharmacy, 700115 Iasi, Romania
3 Discipline of Periodontology, Department of Odontology–Periodontology and Fixed Prosthodontics, Faculty of Dental Medicine, Grigore T. Popa University of Medicine and Pharmacy, 700115 Iasi, Romania
4 Discipline of Dental Technology, Department of Implantology, Removable Dentures, Dental Technology, Faculty of Dental Medicine, Grigore T. Popa University of Medicine and Pharmacy, 700115 Iasi, Romania
5 Discipline of Pediatric Surgery and Orthopedics, 2nd Department of Surgery, Faculty of Medicine, Grigore T. Popa University of Medicine and Pharmacy, 700115 Iasi, Romania
6 Discipline of Orthodontics and Dental-Facial Orthopedics, Department of Surgery, Faculty of Dental Medicine, Grigore T. Popa University of Medicine and Pharmacy, 700115 Iasi, Romania
7 Discipline of Ergonomics, Department of Implantology, Removable Dentures, Dental Technology, Faculty of Dental Medicine, Grigore T. Popa University of Medicine and Pharmacy, 700115 Iasi, Romania
8 Discipline of Preventive Dentistry, Department of Surgery, Faculty of Dental Medicine, Grigore T. Popa University of Medicine and Pharmacy, 700115 Iasi, Romania
* Correspondence: apostu.alina@umfiasi.ro (A.-M.A.); adrian.doloca@umfiasi.ro (A.D.); sorina.solomon@umfiasi.ro (S.M.S.); Tel.: +40-727773545 (A.-M.A.); +40-721501687 (A.D.); +40-722686333 (S.M.S.)
† These authors contributed equally to this work.

Citation: Tanculescu, O.; Apostu, A.-M.; Doloca, A.; Solomon, S.M.; Diaconu-Popa, D.; Ciongradi, C.I.; Vieriu, R.-M.; Aungurencei, O.; Fatu, A.-M.; Ioanid, N.; et al. Perception of Remote Learning by Fixed Prosthodontic Students at a Romanian Faculty of Dentistry. *Int. J. Environ. Res. Public Health* **2023**, *20*, 3622. https://doi.org/10.3390/ijerph20043622

Academic Editor: Giuseppe Alessandro Scardina

Received: 30 December 2022
Revised: 13 February 2023
Accepted: 14 February 2023
Published: 17 February 2023

Abstract: The COVID-19 pandemic has forced the transfer of traditional on-site educational activities to the online environment. This study aimed to evaluate the perception and acceptance of remote learning among fixed prosthodontic students attending the Faculty of Dental Medicine of "Grigore T. Popa" University of Medicine and Pharmacy in Iasi, Romania, and to analyze the feedback regarding their experience with the new online methods, the perceived quality thereof and suggestions for improvement. An observational cross-sectional, online study based on 22 questions was conducted with 259 students. The general opinion of online education was good or very good (40.15%); regarding its efficiency, 28.57% found it efficient while 34.36% found it inefficient or very inefficient; regarding the pleasure of learning online, 45.95% of students enjoyed online learning, while 36.64% did not enjoy it. The problem that was most cited by respondents was that of keeping all students motivated and involved (65.6%). Sixty-two percent of the respondents believe that online dental education should not exist, or just to a small extent, a result justified by the practical nature of the profession. The general opinion was that health risks should be managed and mitigated by using a hybrid system that would allow students to do on-site clinical training with direct contact with patients.

Keywords: dental education; remote learning; online learning; COVID-19; practical skills

1. Introduction

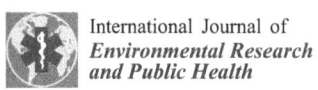

WHO Director-General Tedros Adhanom Ghebreyesus declared, on 30 January 2020, the global outbreak of novel coronavirus to be a public health emergency of international concern (PHEIC) [1], the WHO's highest level of alarm. On 11 March 2020 he declared that the rapidly spreading coronavirus should be considered a pandemic [2,3]. On 13 March 2020, Europe had already become the epicenter of the pandemic, with more reported cases and deaths than the rest of the world combined, apart from the People's Republic of China [4]. Since then, due to the nature of the coronavirus, the entire world has experienced an unprecedented situation, with huge impacts on education and on health systems. The physical distancing and movement restriction of people has become the norm all around the world [5], consecutively impacting universities, regardless of the study programs [6–8]. Thus, the most common measure has been to transfer on-site classes to emergency remote teaching and, in some particular cases, online learning [9], keeping the students in protected environments until the pandemic conditions allow a safe return to face-to-face classes [10–12]. Though learning through online systems is not completely new, this sudden paradigm shift came with the need for a rapid and sustained adaptation for both students and faculty staff [12,13].

For dental faculties in particular, this change meant the transposition of practical work, performed on real patients, into the online environment. Dentistry requires close proximity of the doctor to the patient's mouth, during therapeutic maneuvers, that generate aerosols which are incriminated in virus spreading [14–19]. Consequently, The US Centers for Disease Control and Prevention (CDC) declared dental care-related aerosols and droplets as high risk, considering the apparent resemblance between these aerosols and those specific to medical maneuvers, such as anesthesia or tracheal and nasopharyngeal procedures [15,20]. Therefore, the National Health Commission of China (NHCC), National Health Service of England and American Dental Association (ADA), followed by other dental health regulatory bodies, recommended dental care only in emergency situations during the COVID-19 outbreak period [21,22].

In this context, the dental educators scrambled to adjust an education of a practical and skill-based nature to the online environment. Though various platforms and methods are available for online teaching [23], many of these are of limited use or cannot be employed in the area of dental education [24,25].

For theoretical training, collaboration tools as Microsoft Teams® (Washington, DC, USA, Microsoft Corporation), Zoom® (San Jose, CA, USA, Zoom Video Communications, Inc.), Jitsi® (Campbell, CA, USA, 8 × 8 Inc.), WebEx® (San Jose, CA, USA, Cisco Systems, Inc.) and Moodle® (Perth, Australia, Moodle HQ) were adopted by many universities, for conferences and lectures [23]. The major challenge was the practical preclinical and clinical dental training, for which some limited options are available including virtual reality-based technology, virtual patients, and dental training mannequins, all of which may be supported by lecture-based learning (LBL), problem-based learning (PBL), case-based learning (CBL), team-based learning (TBL), and research-based learning (RBL) [26–28]. Despite the general effort, there has been a high level of concern regarding the impact of these changes on student instruction [29].

In Romania, the bachelor's degree of dentistry (B.D.S) program comprises six years of formal education and is divided into two parts i.e., a pre-clinical training stage (first and second year) and a clinical training stage (third to sixth year). Training programs in dental clinical skills are woven longitudinally into the preclinical curricula starting with the third year, when the students begin to work in clinical environments, on real patients, under the supervision of specialist doctors. Thus, the third and the fourth year are considered the beginning of clinical training and the fifth and the sixth year are the final years of study, consisting predominantly of clinical activities. Grigore T. Popa University of Medicine and Pharmacy of Iasi (UMPh Iasi) is a higher education institution, comprising four faculties: Medicine, Pharmacy, Dental Medicine and Biomedical Engineering. The faculties of Medicine and Dental Medicine have Romanian, English and French programs [30].

On 16 March 2020, the UMPh Iasi announced that all classes would be conducted completely online and remotely, with the cancellation of all on-campus learning, and hands-on and clinical training. The online content of courses and labs was available on the existing e-learning platform of the university. Microsoft Teams® was implemented at the institution level for sending didactic material, conducting classroom conferences and lectures, posting videos, assigning tasks and assessments, and ensuring communication between students and professors. Customized online exams were used, with final hands-on assessment removed.

The 2020–2021 university year was hybrid—the courses being online and the labs on-site (Figure 1), keeping the clinical training on real patients at a minimum. This took into account the existing risk of infection through the various mutations of the virus, despite the high vaccination coverage among the students and teachers [31].

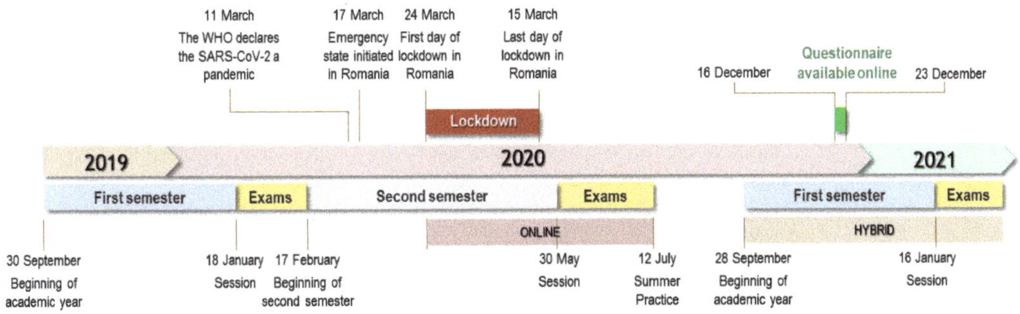

Figure 1. Timeline of academic activity due to the pandemic.

Fixed prosthodontics is one of the main fields of dentistry. At the UMPh Iasi, for the third, fourth and sixth-year students it is a leading compulsory subject of 7, 8 and 5 European Credit Transfer System (ECTS)points, respectively (344 teaching hours).

Modern dental education needs to keep up with the constantly growing knowledge in the biomedical sciences field and involves real-life situations, interpersonal interactions with patients, practice-based learning and the gaining of clinical experience. These are the main pillars of the curricular for dental clinical disciplines aiming to improve students' psychomotor skills and knowledge in diagnosis and treatment option and planning.

In Romania, as in many other countries [23,28,32–36] during the pandemic period, concerns were raised regarding clinical internships at dental clinics [19,37,38]. Clinical training was deeply affected and each medical specialization, including fixed prosthodontics, tried to cope and to find solutions for knowledge transfer and for the compensation for the lack of clinical skills training.

The aim of this study was to evaluate the perception and acceptance of remote learning among fixed prosthodontic students attending our Faculty of Dental Medicine, and to analyze the feedback regarding their experience with the new online methods, the perceived quality thereof and suggestions for improvement.

2. Materials and Methods

2.1. New Teaching Methods

Microsoft Teams is a digital platform that centralizes content, assignments and communication tools in one place. MS Teams is well suited as a university-level virtual environment for education. It engages students with virtual face-to-face communication and activities, and, during the pandemic, it was the next best thing to classical onsite training.

In the first step, the university IT department created MS Teams accounts for all the students and the teaching staff. In this phase, several training sessions were organized so that everyone involved could quickly get familiar with the basic features of MS Teams and could start using the platform for daily educational activities (creating teams, assigning students, uploading content, creating meetings, creating assignments etc.). The selection of this collaboration platform was made based on the features that it offers, but also on the fact that the existing university IT infrastructure is also Microsoft-based and, as such, the integration was a natural process. The adoption of this new educational tool by the students was also a quick and easy process, as MS Teams has some resemblance to the already popular Skype. Members of the teaching staff were given the responsibility to create the necessary teams, mimicking the already existing student group structure and series. MS Teams is complementary to the existing university e-learning platform which provides not only learning content to the students but is, at the same time, an education management tool which registers attendance, student grades, announcements, notifications etc.

2.2. Sample and Questionnaire

An observational cross-sectional, questionnaire-based online survey regarding the remote learning system in use during the COVID-19 pandemic was conducted during 16 December and 23 December 2020. The study focused on students that were supposed to undergo clinical training at a fixed prosthodontics clinic, but the pandemic context drastically limited direct contact between them, the patients and all other persons involved in the educational process. These were students in the third, the fourth and the sixth year of study at the Romanian section of the Faculty of Dental Medicine at the Grigore T. Popa University of Medicine and Pharmacy Iasi.

The questionnaire was created in Romanian and was setup using Google Forms (Mountain View, CA, USA, Alphabet). Misleading questions, multiple negations or unclear formulations were completely avoided. The questionnaire was reviewed for face validity by three experts in dental medical education in order to identify relevant key issues for dental medical students and to assess its relevance and accuracy. Additionally, the study was validated in a pilot study on 32 students. Their feedback and suggestions were used for improvement of the survey. None of these students participated in the final study.

The invitation to participate in the survey and the link to the Google Forms informed consent and questionnaire documents were posted online in Microsoft Teams, in all three teams corresponding to the involved clinical years, for all 488 Romanian students [39].

The representative sample size for the total number of third, fourth and sixth-year students ($n = 488$) was calculated for a confidence level of $p = 95\%$, $z = 1.96$, and margin of error of 5%. The resulting calculated sample size was 216 [40]. Six hundred fifty students were enrolled in the clinical training years (third to sixth year). For the same confidence level ($p = 95\%$) and margin of error (5%) the calculated sample size was 242. The questionnaire was answered by 259 students, representing 53% of the total number for the three targeted years. The sample was also representative for all clinical training years.

Participant sampling was volunteer based, and no incentives were used for study participation. All respondents delivered answers to all questions in the questionnaire, making the acquired data valid and usable as provided. No data were eliminated.

The questionnaire focused on students' perceptions and feedback on didactic activities during pandemic period and was structured into three parts. The first part included single and multiple-choice general questions regarding remote learning and its impact (Q1–Q12). The second part also included multiple-choice questions related to the perceived quality of remote teaching, learning and assessment in the fixed prosthodontics disciplines for both theoretical knowledge and practical skills (Q13–Q20). Finally, the third part included two open questions, asking for suggestions to improve didactic activity for fixed prosthodontics disciplines and also for free comments on this subject.

The first eight questions (Q1–Q8) had answers rated on a five-point Likert scale, representing ordinal variables, with different constructions of the answers, and each question was attached to the response scale with the corresponding coding. The response categories for these questions are presented in Table 1. The lower the score, the stronger is the negative perception of the student and the higher the score, the stronger is the positive students' perceptions and acceptance of remote learning and its consequences.

Table 1. The response categories for questions one to eight.

Questions	Answers Rank				
	1	2	3	4	5
Q1. What do you think about online education?	very bad	bad	neutral	good	very good
Q2. How efficient is online education for you?	not at all	a little bit	medium	a lot	very much
Q3. Do you enjoy learning online?	not at all	not really	neutral	yes, but with some changes	yes, definitely
Q4. To what extent did the relationship with colleagues suffer?	very much	a lot	moderate	a little bit	not at all
Q5. To what extent has the relationship with the teaching staff suffered?	very much	a lot	moderate	a little bit	not at all
Q6. To what extent do you receive help from teachers during your online study?	very much	a lot	moderate	a little bit	not at all
Q7. To what extent have the changes in the last 10 months affected you psychologically?	very much	a lot	moderate	a little bit	not at all
Q8. In your opinion, after the end of the pandemic period, should online teaching remain a component of dental education?	no	to littleextent	moderate extent	to a largeextent	yes

The questions 9–20 (Q9–Q20) were purely nominal, with no ranking of the possible answers, while the remaining two were open-ended questions (Q21, Q22).

2.3. *Statistical Study*

In the first stage of the statistical analysis, the construction validity was tested using factors and reliability analysis, i.e., Cronbach's alpha test. Descriptive statistical methods were used, determining frequencies for categorical responses and the distribution diagrams of these responses.

The interrelation between some categorical variables was analyzed using contingency tables. To check if there is a statistically significant relationship between these variables, a chi-square test was performed. To assess the strength of the relationship, for ordinal variables, the Spearman's rank correlation coefficient was determined. For nominal variables, the strength of the association was analyzed using Cramer's V.

The answers to the open-ended questions were evaluated qualitatively and if there were more than two similar statements then they were placed into groups. This helped to understand the student needs and prioritize the measures needed to improve the quality of e-teaching and e-learning.

Data analysis was carried out using IBM SPSS Statistics, version 28 (IBM, Armonk, NY, USA). Statistical significance was set at $p = 0.05$.

3. Results

3.1. *Student Perception and Feedback on Remote Learning and Its Impact*

The compilation of the questions and their internal consistency (Q1–Q8) was tested and the reliability for each latent variable used in this study was confirmed by Cronbach's alpha test ($\alpha = 0.829$). Table 2 shows the parallel correlations between the variables, which are generally weak, with only six correlations above 0.500.

Table 2. Spearman's rank correlation coefficient for Q1–Q8 (N of valid cases = 259).

		Q1	Q2	Q3	Q4	Q5	Q6	Q7	Q8
Q1	χ^2	-							
	ρ	1							
	1-β	-							
Q2	χ^2	285.979	-						
	ρ	0.786 **	1						
	1-β	1	-						
Q3	χ^2	230.655	210.226	-					
	ρ	0.635 **	0.708 **	1					
	1-β	1	1	-					
Q4	χ^2	44.846	40.859	33.992	-				
	ρ	0.234 **	0.306 **	0.229 **	1				
	1-β	0.883	0.991	0.866	-				
Q5	χ^2	69.652	118.120	69.142	192.041	-			
	ρ	0.418 **	0.490 **	0.359 **	0.586 **	1			
	1-β	1	1	0.999	1	-			
Q6	χ^2	53.662	63.246	33.946	29.172	39.950	-		
	ρ	0.386 **	0.375 **	0.236 **	0.189 **	0.288 **	1		
	1-β	1	1	0.889	0.677	0.981	-		
Q7	χ^2	51.571	72.787	50.956	57.135	57.083	48.482	-	
	ρ	0.334 **	0.421 **	0.330 **	0.332 **	0.358 **	0.318 **	1	
	1-β	0.998	1	0.997	0.997	0.999	0.995	-	
Q8	χ^2	99.090	97.099	113.490	18.962	40.878	18.202	38.243	-
	ρ	0.493 **	0.536 **	0.590 **	0.168 **	0.282 **	0.063	0.230 **	1
	1-β	1	1	1	0.547	0.976	0.059	0.869	-

$\chi2$ = Pearson's chi-squared statistic for df = 16; ρ = Spearman's rank correlation coefficient; 1-β = statistical power of the test. ** Correlation is significant at the 0.01 level (two-tailed).

The first three questions are related to the students' general opinion about online education (Q1), their perception about its efficiency (Q2) and the pleasure of learning online (Q3). One hundred four students (40.15%) have a good or a very good opinion about online education (Q1), while 99 (38.22%) are neutral and 56 (21.62%) have a bad or very bad opinion about online learning. Regarding the efficiency (Q2), only 74 (28.57%) found online learning to be efficient, while 89 (34.36%) found it efficient or very efficient. Of the students, 45.95% (119) enjoy online learning, while 36.64% (95) do not enjoy it (Q3) (Figure 2). Pearson's chi-squared tests showed a strong correlation between the three items (Q1, Q2 and Q3) ($p < 0.001$) (Table 2).

Fifty-eight (22.4%) participants stated that their relationship with their colleagues suffered considerably, a percentage to which we add those who felt a moderate alteration of their relationship (29.3%) (Q4). It seems that not only the relations with colleagues have suffered but also those with the teaching staff (Q5). Fifty-six, 4% of the participants in the study claimed that this type of relationship suffered, from a moderate to an extreme intensity, especially in the conditions in which 17.4% of students perceived the support that they received from their teacher to be absent or very reduced (Q6). However, at the same time, the vast majority (81.9%) of students regard the help from teaching staff as moderate to extremely helpful. Of the students, 35.2% were not psychologically affected at all or only slightly affected, while 37.1% perceived moderate psychological changes (Q7). Having the experience of all types of learning—exclusively onsite, exclusively online and hybrid—62% of the respondents believe that online education should not exist, or just to a small extent, a result justified by the practical nature of the profession and by the university profile (Q8) (Figure 1).

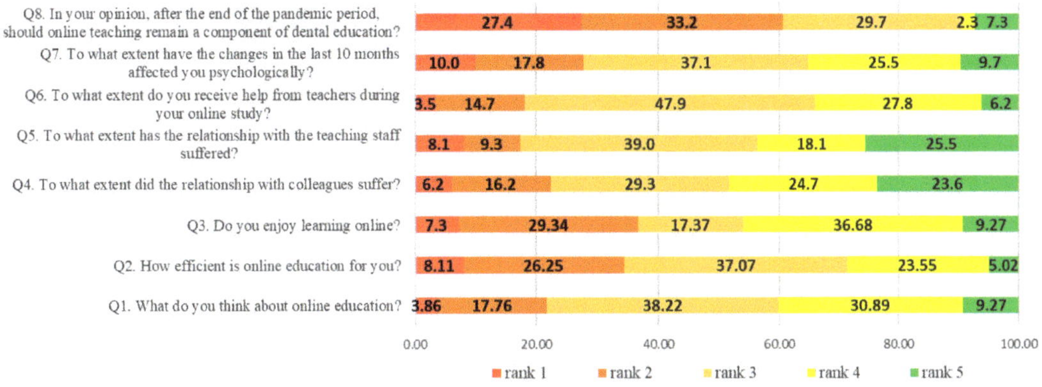

Figure 2. Distribution of relative frequencies of answers to questions one to three (Q1–Q8). The numbers in the bars indicate the percentages of the answers received (n = 259).

Q9 focused on the possible motivations for enjoying online/remote learning. The respondents were pleasantly surprised primarily by the high degree of flexibility offered by this type of education (63.6%), its ease of use (48.2%) and the accessibility of platforms, materials and resources (45.1%) (Figure 3).

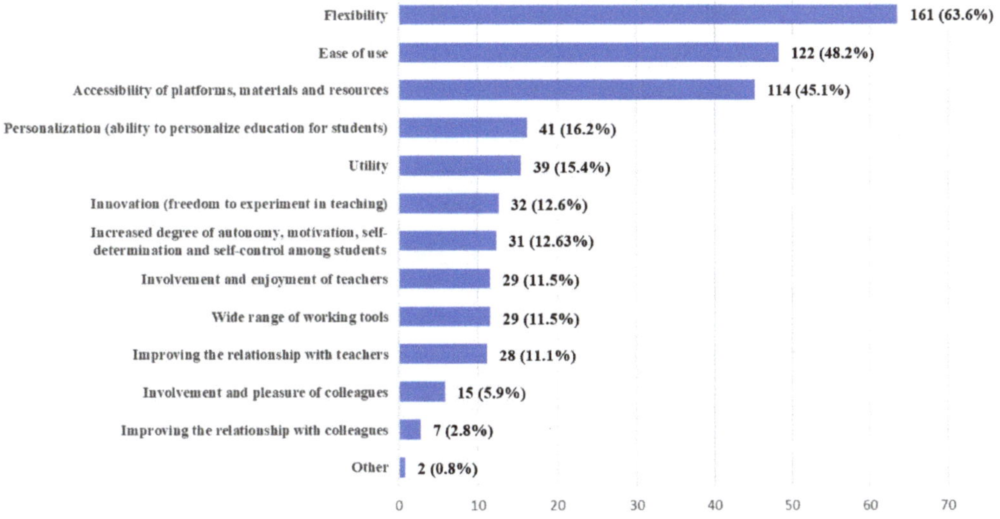

Figure 3. Frequency distribution of answers to question 9 (Q9): "What has pleasantly surprised you about online/remote learning?". The numbers in the bars indicate the counts and the percentages of the answers (n = 259).

The transition to online/remote learning (Q10), in addition to the need for immediate implementation, has encountered several other obstacles. According to the majority of dental students, the main challenges that were encountered were keeping all the students motivated and involved (65.6%) and the practical nature of the discipline (54.4%) (Figure 4).

The low level of digital pedagogical competence of the teachers and the difficulty of translating the practical training to the online environment, were two other important obstacles claimed by the students.

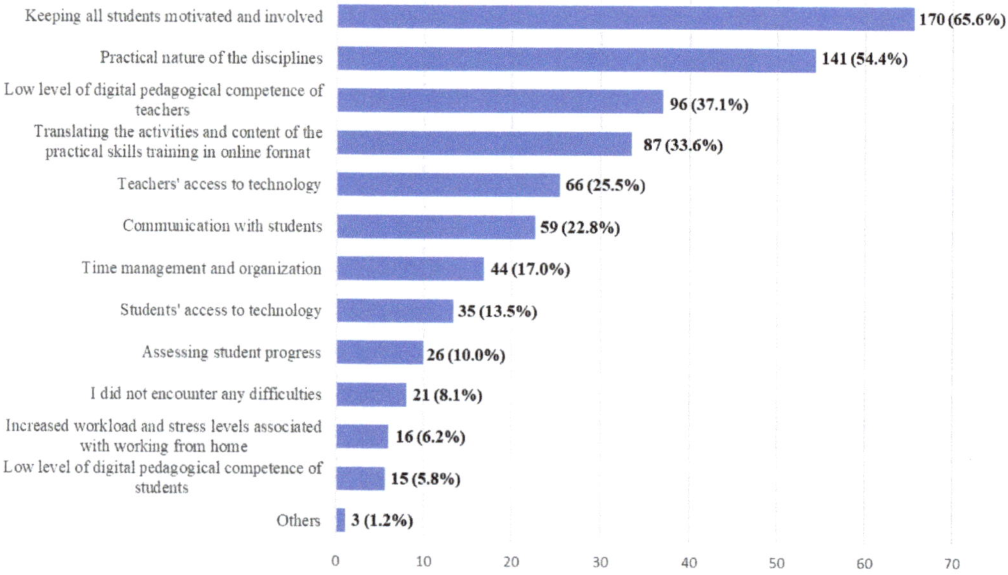

Figure 4. Frequency distribution of answers to question 10 (Q10): "In your opinion, what were the main obstacles to the transition to online/remote learning? Select up to five options". The numbers indicate the counts and the percentages of the answers (n = 259).

More than half of the students (56.4%) found the quality of the presentation to be the main instrument to increase student involvement during online/remote activities (Q11). The clinical and practical training component of the discipline is another factor which motivates the students to stay involved and focused (49%), followed by the quality of the information itself (44%) and an increase in the level of interaction between the students and the teacher (41.3%) (Figure 5).

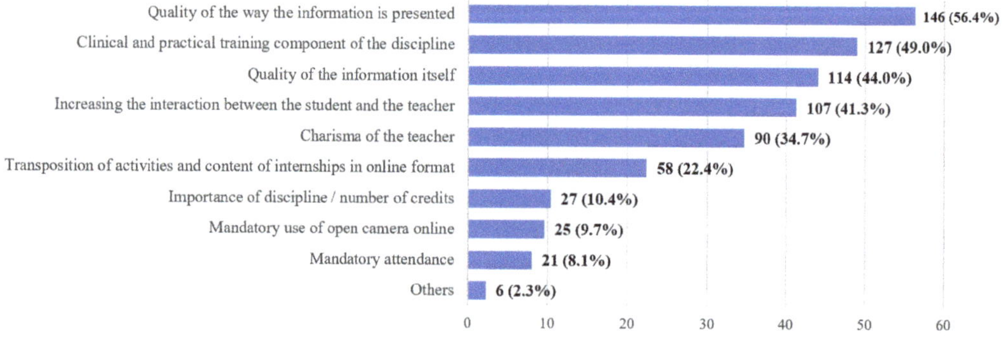

Figure 5. Frequency distribution of answers to Q11: "In your opinion what could increase your involvement during online activities?". The numbers indicate the counts and the percentages of the answers (n = 259).

Of the students, 74.5% are convinced that dental education will be changed due to the COVID-19 crisis (Q12) (Figure 6).

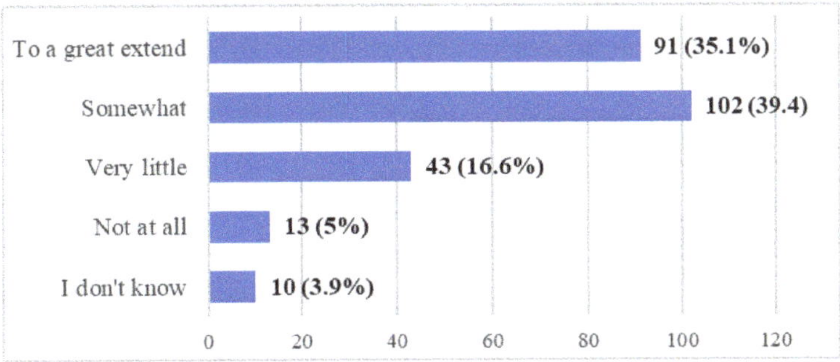

Figure 6. Frequency distribution of answers to Q12: "In your opinion, will the COVID-19 crisis change the future of dental education?". The numbers indicate the counts and the percentages of the answers (n = 259).

3.2. Student Perception and Feedback on Remote Teaching, Learning and Assessment at the Fixed Prosthodontics Disciplines for Both Theoretical Knowledge and Practical Skills

The major challenge related to online teaching has been the conveying of practical notions and clinical procedures to students, activities that traditionally require the presence of a patient. However, equally, we were interested in students' opinions on the theoretical aspects of the courses, in terms of the manner of presentation—online, onsite or hybrid—and the personal interactions with the academic staff.

Regarding the preference for teaching theoretical notions—online, onsite or hybrid (Q13)—the respondents have equally divided opinions between hybrid and online. In the case of the online version, they prefer an increased share of activities carried out synchronously, with real-time interaction with the teaching staff. In their opinion, the teacher should personally present the course and thus reduce the need to watch recordings or video demonstrations with pre-recorded explanations (Q14) (60.23%) (Table 3).

Table 3. Spearman's rank correlation coefficient for Q1–Q8 (N of valid cases = 259).

		Q13-Do You Consider That the Teaching of Theoretical Notions Should Be Done:								
	Answer Options	**Hybrid**	**Online**	**Onsite**	χ^2	*df*	ϕ_c	*p*	**Total**	
		N	N	N					N	%
Q14	Increasing the amount of asynchronous content	34	50	19	7, 873	2	0.17	<0.020	103	39.77
	Increasing the amount of synchronous content	65	49	42					156	60.23
	Total N	99	99	61					259	
	Total %	38.22	38.22	23.55						100.00

Q14 = Do you think that the following should be considered when teaching theoretical notions online

N = count; $\chi 2$ = Pearson's chi-squared statistic; ϕ_c = Cramer's V coefficient; p = p-value.

A very large proportion of students also desired (Q15) the inclusion, along with the pure theoretical notions, of a greater number of video demonstrations of diagnostic and treatment methods (74.9%), as well as an increased share of clinical cases (68.34%), with more active involvement of students during the course (36.29%) (Figure 7).

Regarding the practical notions (Q16), there is an obvious preference for teaching using real patients, in a proportion of 100% (46.72%), or 25% theoretically and 75% on real and/or virtual patients (48.65%) (Figure 8).

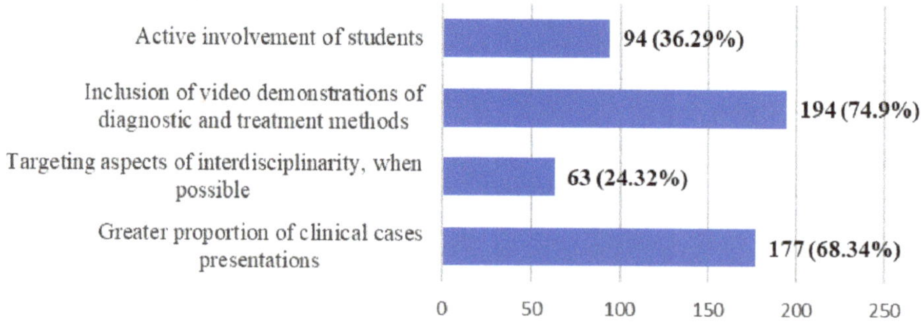

Figure 7. Frequency distribution of answers to Q15: "Do you consider that in teaching the theoretical notions the following should be considered:". The numbers indicate the counts and the percentages of the answers (n = 259).

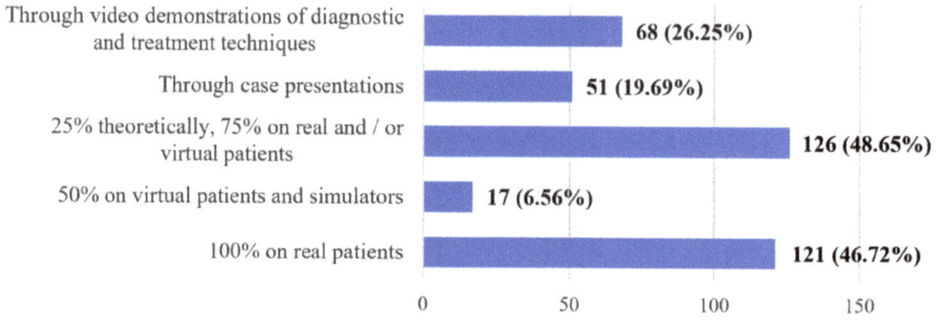

Figure 8. Frequency distribution of answers to Q16: "Do you consider that the teaching of practical knowledge should be carried out:". The numbers indicate the counts and the percentages of the answers (n = 259).

Most students (72.97%) prefer the following sequence of steps in the learning process (Q17): teaching, individual study and discussions (Figure 9).

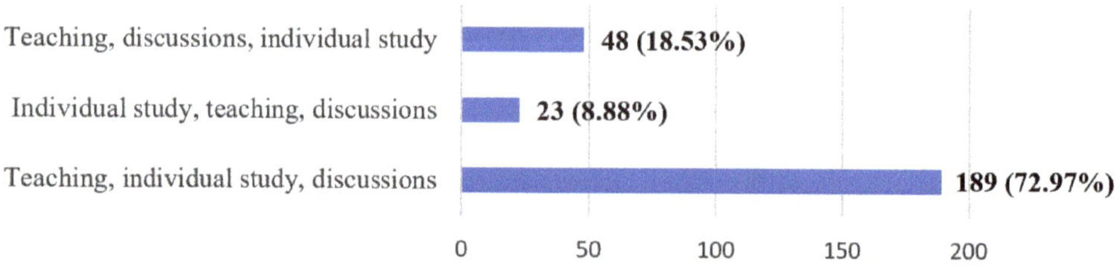

Figure 9. Frequency distribution of answers to Q17: "What do you think should be the sequence of steps?". The numbers indicate the counts and the percentages of the answers (n = 259).

Q18 is related to the factors that could increase the quality of the clinical training considering the online conditions. The main factor is clear and understandable content (91.89%), along with a specifying of the practical usefulness and relevance of the received information (57.92%) (Figure 10).

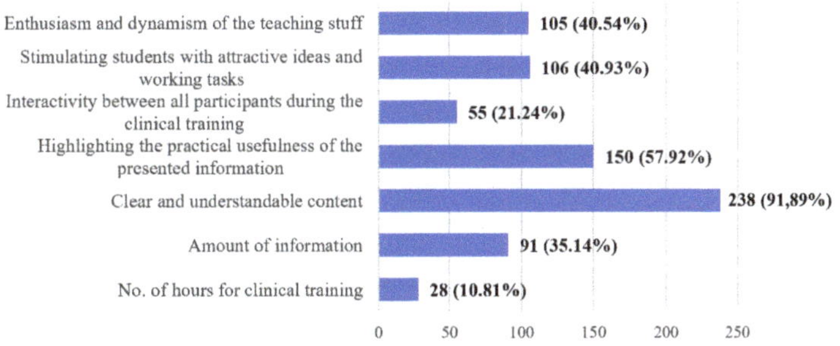

Figure 10. Frequency distribution of answers to Q18. "What are, in your opinion, the top three factors that influence the quality of clinical training?". The numbers indicate the counts and the percentages of the answers (n = 259).

According to the students, the best way to facilitate the assimilation of the transmitted practical and theoretical notions (Q19) is through discussions and debates based on clinical situations (61.00%) (Figure 11).

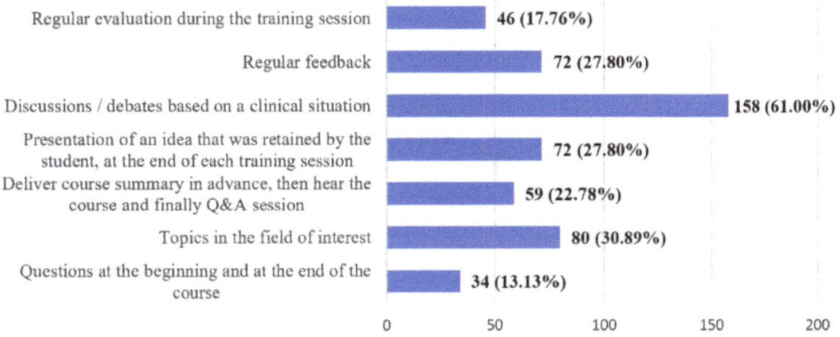

Figure 11. Frequency distribution of answers to Q19: "What are, in your opinion, the most appropriate methods for the optimal assimilation of the conveyed practical and theoretical notions?". The numbers indicate the counts and the percentages of the answers (n = 259).

Regarding the most popular method of examination/evaluation for disciplines with a practical component (Q20), students would prefer onsite examination (58.3%), with the performing of practical maneuvers (52.51%) and, in smaller proportion, the simple and multiple choices tests (31.27%), or use of virtual patients (29.34%) (Figure 12).

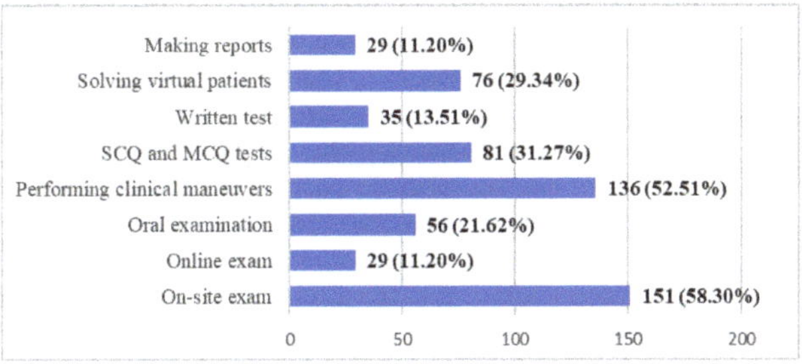

Figure 12. Frequency distribution of answers to Q20: "What are, in your opinion, the most appropriate evaluation methods, for the predominant practical/applied disciplines?". The numbers indicate the counts and the percentages of the answers (n = 259).

3.3. Open-Ended Questions–Students' Suggestions and Opinions on Didactic Activity at the Fixed Prosthodontics Disciplines

The responses to open-ended questions (Q21: "What suggestions do you have for improving the teaching activity? Specify which of the disciplines you are making the recommendations for" and Q22: "Additional comments are welcome. Please note them down") revealed the strengths and the limitations of online learning and some of the concerns and suggestions of our students, related to this new teaching approach (Table 4).

Table 4. Some of the most relevant student opinions.

Strengths	Limitations	Concerns	Suggestions
Unlike previous years, we managed to attend all the courses. More time to spend in a familiar, safe environment. Reduced costs for transportation and accommodation for students from outside the university center. Increased usage of digital teaching content during the classes. Availability of online teaching materials to be watched at any time.	Lack of practical skills. Dentistry is not a theoretical domain; hands-on practical training is mandatory. We were struggling to keep our concentration and motivation at a high level. Lack of interactivity with the peers and teaching staff. Not all the disciplines allow the courses to be recorded and do not offer online materials. Lack of separation between the work environment and home environment. Distraction by family-related issues in the home environment. Internet connectivity issues.	Because of the lack of practical activity, the information will be superficially assimilated, without a deep understanding. Lack of experience of patient interaction and treatment, with concerns about the future profession. Lack of social interaction and the alteration of the student–professor relationship. Stress and uncertainty related to the new online examination method, irrelevant and altered quality of online examination. Losing the privacy of one's own home because of the need to turn on the camera and bringing the stress related to the faculty activities to the private environment at home.	In person attendance at the clinical training. The level of interactivity during the online classes should be increased. On-site examination. At least those who had COVID should attend on-site classes.

Some of the most frequent comments related to the strength points were the high attendance of online lectures, with the possibility of spending more time in a safe environment with family and with lower costs. The accessibility of digital content not otherwise available in the classrooms is perceived as an improvement to the teaching process. The most critical observation was that dental education is inherently an activity that must develop practical skills and cannot be performed only at a theoretical level or without any direct contact with the patient. Another frequent problem claimed by the students is the difficulty of keeping their focus and motivation to get involved during the online lectures. From these statements some concerns are derived, including insufficient abilities and training in patient treatment, and insufficient knowledge of the new online assessment method. The common suggestion for improving the educational process was to switch back to on-site teaching. Online teaching is accepted as a temporary solution given the pandemic situation, but one that is not suited for permanent adoption because of the many disadvantages. These ideas are summarized in one of the students' answers: "I consider myself one of those focused and engaged students and I've still had classes to which I couldn't pay attention at all. I don't think the problem is the professor. They all worked very hard. The problem is that it is done online."

4. Discussion

Due to its high level of transmissibility and casualties and to the imposed restrictions associated with it, the COVID-19 pandemic has disrupted almost every area of human activity. Education, which relies on people getting together to share knowledge, has been especially affected, making most of the usual activities impossible. Despite all these restrictions and challenges, dental schools around the world have quickly and creatively adapted to the new situation, to ensure continuity of the educational processes [11–13,19,38,41,42]. Grigore T. Popa University of Medicine and Pharmacy Iasi, similar to other universities, already had a digital platform that supported day –to-day academic activities: digital material sharing, management of absences and exam results, teaching staff evaluations, etc. However, the platform neither supported real-time communication between students and teaching staff, nor real-time management of the student periodic evaluations. This means that students were accustomed to the digital platform, mainly for administrative tasks, but the educational component was 100% a traditional one, with lectures given in amphitheaters and practical activities that took place in clinics. Therefore, the accelerated transition to a new, online way of teaching and evaluating was a huge challenge, both for teaching staff and for students [12,13].

Even if these days, the pandemic seems to be fading, we must recognize that the gains in the usage of new digital technologies and new teaching methods are expected to continue even after the pandemic is over [41,43,44]. Most of the dental schools have already made the transition back to face-to-face teaching, but the new methods used during the pandemic can and should complete and enhance the classical approach [45,46].

Our study is focused on the fixed prosthodontics disciplines and students, highlighting the needs and expectations for this domain.

Looking at the frequency distributions of answers provided to the Likert scale questions, we can extract a few interesting insights. Most of the answers are in the middle of the scale, avoiding very bad and very good statements. This is due to the realization that we are dealing with an exceptional situation, and we are trying to cope with it, doing our best. As an exception, answers to questions about the extent to which the relationships with the colleagues and with the teaching staff were affected, had a higher frequency towards the favorable end of the scale, stating that they were not at all affected. This is mainly due to the fact that, even prior to the pandemic, a lot of digital communication tools were available and which students used privately: Skype, WhatsApp, Messenger, etc. This ensured that they could stay in contact and not suffer from total isolation. These findings are also supported by a recent study made in different dental schools in the European region [47]. In addition to this, given the potential for psychological problems among students and academic staff induced by personal, social, emotional and academic situations [6,12,33,46,48,49], the Grigore T. Popa University of Medicine and Pharmacy Iasi offered guidance and emotional support on its online platform, via professional counseling sessions [33,50,51].

Another question with a high frequency of answers, this time towards the unfavorable end of the scale, is about the remaining online teaching methods after the end of the pandemic period. This clear negative reaction was caused not only by the difficulties posed by the new online teaching method and the new tools that have to be used, but also by the fact that without direct contact with patients and without hands-on practice, the quality of the educational process will significantly decrease [11,12,36,43,52,53]. In this regard, the biggest challenge for lecturers and professors has been to compensate for the lack of clinical training, and to re-invent and re-adapt the educational process in a very short period of time, without any previous preparation or planning, and while also constrained by distance, legal and ethical problems (such as the use of "show and share" patient clinical pictures in digital environment) [23,36].

When it comes to the positive sides of online teaching and learning, students have appreciated the flexibility, the ease of use and the potential for innovation. This shows that the introduction of new technologies and digital tools was not, by any means, a problem, but something that students embraced with lightness although it required some effort on their part as shown in our research and reported in different other studies [11,12,36,52,54,55].

If we were to pinpoint just one major issue linked to the transition to online/remote learning, this would be the lack of motivation and involvement in activities performed online. This aspect shows up numerous times through the questionnaire and seems to be the main hurdle affecting the new way of working during the pandemic [23,33,36]. Based on the experience of teaching staff with online lectures, an increased student attendance is not necessarily relevant, if their focus and engagement are low or, in some cases, even very low. Lack of visual contact with students, interference of home-related activities and interaction with family members, and difficulty in setting clear boundaries between the personal and professional space and schedules, usually account for disruptions of students' concentration on the presented topics and for low engagement levels [48]. Our study tried to further investigate the ways in which this problem could be alleviated, and the possible solutions indicated by the students revolve around the quality of the presentations, the level of interaction between students and educators and around the possibility of more focus on the clinical and practical aspects of the presented information.

Given the pluses and minuses of the online/remote didactic activities, the majority (75%) of the participants in this study expressed their belief that the future of dental education will be impacted by the COVID-19 crisis. This is a general belief that has been revealed by many studies [9,10,12,23,29,36,42,44–46,48,50,53,54,56].

The type of teaching (hybrid/online/onsite) of the theoretical notions in relation to the content type was another evaluated issue. The outcome underlines the preference for online or hybrid teaching, with the distinction between the two being decided by the type of content—synchronous or asynchronous. The correlation between the two variables is a significant one. This is somehow expected because synchronous content requires real-time interaction with the teaching staff, while asynchronous content can be delivered fully online, without the instant supervision of an educator [36,57]. Overall, the students were more favorable to direct interaction with the professor, as it provides an opportunity to ask questions in real time and to get instant feedback [57,58]. In analyzing the online teaching of theoretical notions, the respondents identified two main possible ways of ensuring higher quality: using video demonstrations of diagnostic and treatment methods and including a higher proportion of clinical cases in the delivered presentations. These measures could, at least partly, compensate for the reduced level of interaction between the students and the educators and patients in the online environment.

Regarding the asynchronous teaching/learning, due to technological advancements and several undeniable benefits, dental podcasts have become popular among students and practitioners as tools for learning and for updating knowledge in general. Some studies [59] have shown that, in comparison with text book reading, watching video podcasts is a more efficient learning method, an efficiency that is reflected by higher scores in MCQ tests. Short-duration podcasts in particular [60] were perceived by students as useful supplementary learning tools that aided them for revision and in their preparation for assessments. An in-depth analysis of the importance of podcasts in learning in the medical field was undertaken by [61].

The value brought by this kind of teaching/learning practice is founded on several benefits that relate to the new modern way of living and working:

a. flexibility—being disconnected from the creation and transmission of the training material, the trainee can access it at any time, any place and using the preferred device. After downloading the material, some or all of the content can be played at the student's discretion, so as to facilitate the learning process.
b. engagement—the content is more engaging than the mere reading of a textbook, further supporting the learning process.
c. wide accessibility—the content can be accessed anywhere in the world, thus reaching a much wider audience compared with on-site delivered lectures.

Regarding the teaching of practical skills, the general opinion is that this should be undertaken more on real patients and be less reliant on the use of video demonstrations and virtual patients. This is again linked to the fact that dentistry is regarded as a practical domain that should deliver education in a very practical way and in a setting that is as close as possible to a real clinical environment. Other alternatives are regarded as moving away from the normal path that education should progress on and could be accepted only because of the exceptional situation generated by the COVID-19 pandemic.

Though there is no replacement for hands-on clinical experience, versatile and immersive learning experiences can be obtained through haptic technologies and virtual (Moog Simodent) and augmented reality (DentSim, CDS-100, IRIS) [62]. These have the potential to deliver relevant, flexible, and immersive learning experiences if they are further enhanced according to the needs of dentistry. At the same time, they should be portable and affordable for large-scale usage by students [10,24,43–45,54]. Meanwhile, for medicine, some applications and software that are focused on complex, clinically based scenarios are available for use in virtual group discussions to improve students' decision-making and diagnostic skills [26,63]. However, for dentistry in general, and prosthodontics, in particular, there are few options available for students [27].

Artificial intelligence (AI) is being increasingly adopted in the field of dentistry, including dental education. While other technologies, such as robotics, are expensive and require a certain environment in which to operate, AI can be delivered at much lower costs and to a wider range of students. AI can be used to provide virtual simulations of dental procedures, allowing students to practice and improve their skills in a safe and controlled environment. This can help mitigate the risk of errors or failures during real-life procedures.

Regarding the sequence of the learning activities, most of the respondents opted for teaching, individual study and discussions. The students considered it more opportune for the student–instructor and student–student interactions/discussions to be taken after the lecture series and individual study. This sets a high priority on individual study with the possibility to clear up some difficult subjects during discussions with members of the teaching staff [58].

Clinical training should be performed using clear and understandable content and focusing on the practical usage of the presented information, engagement of the students in different and attractive tasks, high interactivity between the participants to the study-group, and, not the least, by an enthusiastic and dynamic approach on the part of the professor. At the same time, the optimal assimilation of information should be supported through discussions/debates on relevant clinical situations, as pointed out by the students' answers. Although these responses were not surprising, the implementation of these goals was difficult, the teaching staff were found to be unprepared for the translation of the clinical internships from the actual patient's head to the online environment. It is worth noting that the literature highlights the general dissatisfaction of students regarding the organization of clinical internships, other online options being unable to compensate for the lack of actual practice [34,35,47,64].

The assessments are an important aspect of the educational process and were impacted as well by the pandemic. As educators, we tried to find out what the proper methods of assessment would be, given the challenges imposed by the fight against COVID-19. In our study, most of the respondents chose the on-site examination type, despite the risks related to their health. They opted for clinical maneuvers as a means to evaluate the assimilated knowledge, in the context of on-site evaluation. Simple choice questions (SCQ) and multiple-choice questions (MCQ) were also regarded as a possibility, being methods that are compatible with the available online tools. During the pandemic, universities have adopted several online assessment methods, including MCQ, oral examinations, video oral assessment, essays etc. While these are compatible with digital tools (MS Teams, Skype, Email), other problems arose: identity verification, authorship, and plagiarism, all of which might affect the validity and the relevance of the assessment [33]. Some of the universities or disciplines canceled or postponed the examinations [46], other universities adopted new procedures for the pandemic. Assessment of clinical competences was in some cases done using virtual patients, which could be a digital alternative to the face-to-face examination of clinical abilities. These specifically target assessment of clinical reasoning and of diagnostic skills.

Recent advances in AI have produced systems such as OpenAI's ChatGPT and Google's Bard, based on optimized language models and capable of interacting in a conversational way. This technology offers multiple opportunities for education, but it still must be seen how it can be best applied to specific needs and what adjustments are necessary so that it is used in a responsible way. The main goal is to improve and enhance the learning process while minimizing the risk of plagiarism and fraud related to assignments and exams.

Among the limitations of this research were the way in which the survey was conducted at only one dental institution, the study participants were self-selected and some of the questions focused on fixed prosthodontic disciplines, with clinical skills curricula. Another limitation of this study was the low response rate of the dental students (53%), which may contribute to non-response bias since targeted dental students were underrepresented. Based on the example of one department in the university and one single university in the country, the study cannot be positioned as a reference point for the actual situation. However, the authors consider that sharing experience is important and each university can consistently contribute to a new and improved teaching/learning paradigm. Student feedback is a valuable instrument in shaping curriculum and this is why their perspective and acceptance of the encountered transformations during the pandemic period have been previously reported in many studies [11,12,25,28,34–36,47,55]. Future research should be performed so as to also involve the teaching staff, to reconcile both views regarding the educational process.

At the same time, revolutionary technologies such as robotics and artificial intelligence (AI) could also contribute to the enhancement of the way dental education is delivered [65]. A study that looks at the acceptance and the impact of these novel methods among dental students would be an important tool that might help to integrate them along the traditional teaching practices.

According to the results of this study, clinical training was the major challenge during pandemic crises. Despite the high acceptance of new digital tools, not all students embraced online learning, since there is a need for consistent enhancement of these tools to support clinical training. In the context of the limited availability of virtual or enhanced reality, proper digital tools (virtual reality-based technology, virtual patients, PBL, CBL etc.) can improve clinical reasoning and decision making. Still, for practical skills training, direct contact with the patient is mandatory. None of the other available methods were able to compensate for the lack of practical skills training. During the pandemic we put an accent on clinical reasoning and decision making which was an improvement compared with previous years. In our case, as a consequence of the feedback gained from this study, we had to adjust accordingly and implement, over the following years, the recovery of practical skills training in fixed prosthodontics. Constant feedback from students and flexible curricula structures might be powerful instruments in adapting the educational tools to student needs.

On one hand, the curriculum must be flexible enough to accommodate a wider range of learning tools that include digital applications which can be used, if needed, without a physical presence. On the other hand, it is necessary to expand these tools to stimulate clinical reasoning and decision making remotely, without physical contact. Additionally, for the improvement of dental clinical skills and beyond the traditional simulators, enhanced and virtual reality systems with haptic feedback are required, though these entail high costs and require special equipment.

5. Conclusions

COVID-19 was a global force majeure event that imposed drastic measures on all levels of human existence: healthcare, education, economy, and social life. For dental education in particular, the disruption imposed by this pandemic revealed once more the importance of direct contact of students with teaching staff and with patients. Regardless of the progress in computer technology used for online teaching, there is a unanimous opinion that dentistry is not a domain that can be predominantly taught online. However, online teaching can be a substantial addition to the traditional on-site method. This is due to several advantages that online teaching offers, including: high availability, usage of an enhanced variety of digital materials, independence of location and time, reduced costs for both students and universities. If we are to admit any positive sides of this tragic event, it would be a better understanding of the value of human interrelations and the accelerated progress of medical and computer technology, especially of the online communication platforms, telemedicine, and simulations. These technologies should be integrated into the educational process as an instrument to boost the trainer's ability to engage students and improve their practical skills.

Author Contributions: Conceptualization, O.T., A.-M.A., D.D.-P. and C.I.C.; methodology, O.T., C.I.C., O.A. and C.I.S.; software, A.D., O.A. and C.I.S.; validation, S.M.S., C.I.C., D.D.-P. and R.-M.V.; formal analysis, O.T., A.D. and R.-M.V.; investigation, A.-M.A., O.A., A.-M.F., N.I., M.S. and R.-M.V.; resources, O.A., A.-M.F. and D.D.-P.; data curation, O.T., A.D., S.M.S. and A.-M.F.; writing—original draft preparation, O.T., A.-M.A., N.I. and M.S.; writing—review and editing, O.T., A.-M.A., A.D., A.-M.F. and C.I.S.; visualization, S.M.S., R.-M.V., C.I.C., N.I. and M.S.; supervision, S.M.S., D.D.-P., C.I.C. and C.I.S.; project administration, O.T. and D.D.-P. All authors have read and agreed to the published version of the manuscript.

Funding: This research received no external funding.

Institutional Review Board Statement: The study was conducted in accordance with the Declaration of Helsinki and approved by the Institutional Ethics Committee of Grigore T. Popa University of Medicine and Pharmacy Nr. 269/11.02.2023 for studies involving humans.

Informed Consent Statement: In accordance with the EU General Data Protection Regulations 2016/679, informed consent regarding the analysis of their data was obtained from all subjects involved in the study, before starting the survey. Subjects were informed that the data they share are non-personal and no one will be able to know if they participated in this study.

Data Availability Statement: The data that support the findings of this study are available on request from the corresponding author.

Conflicts of Interest: The authors declare no conflict of interest.

References

1. WHO. WHO Director-General's Statement on IHR Emergency Committee on Novel Coronavirus (2019-nCoV). Available online: https://www.who.int/director-general/speeches/detail/who-director-general-s-statement-on-ihr-emergency-committee-on-novel-coronavirus-(2019-ncov) (accessed on 19 June 2022).
2. WHO. WHO Director-General's Opening Remarks at the Media Briefing on COVID-19. 11 March 2020. Available online: https://www.who.int/director-general/speeches/detail/who-director-general-s-opening-remarks-at-the-media-briefing-on-covid-19---11-march-2020 (accessed on 19 June 2022).
3. WHO. Coronavirus Disease (COVID-19) Pandemic. Available online: https://www.euro.who.int/en/health-topics/health-emergencies/coronavirus-covid-19/novel-coronavirus-2019-ncov (accessed on 19 June 2022).
4. WHO. WHO Director-General's Opening Remarks at the Media Briefing on COVID-19. 13 March 2020. Available online: https://www.who.int/director-general/speeches/detail/who-director-general-s-opening-remarks-at-the-mission-briefing-on-covid-19---13-march-2020 (accessed on 19 June 2022).
5. Painter, M.; Qiu, T. Political Beliefs affect Compliance with Government Mandates. *J. Econ. Behav. Organ. Forthcom.* **2021**, *185*, 688–701. [CrossRef]
6. Cao, W.J.; Fang, Z.W.; Hou, G.Q.; Han, M.; Xu, X.R.; Dong, J.X.; Zheng, J.Z. The psychological impact of the COVID-19 epidemic on college students in China. *Psychiatry Res.* **2020**, *287*, 5. [CrossRef]

7. Wang, C.; Cheng, Z.; Yue, X.-G.; McAleer, M. Risk Management of COVID-19 by Universities in China. *J. Risk Financ. Manag.* **2020**, *13*, 36. [CrossRef]
8. Gaudin, A.; Arbab-Chirani, R.; Pérez, F. Effect of COVID-19 on Dental Education and Practice in France. *Front. Dent. Med.* **2020**, *1*, 5. [CrossRef]
9. Hodges, C.; Moore, S.; Lockee, B.; Trust, T.; Bond, A. The difference between emergency remote teaching and online learning. *Educ. Rev.* **2020**. Available online: https://er.educause.edu/articles/2020/3/the-difference-between-emergency-remote-teaching-and-online-learning (accessed on 19 June 2022).
10. Witze, A. Universities will never be the same after the coronavirus crisis. *Nature* **2020**, *582*, 162–164. [CrossRef]
11. Butnaru, G.I.; Niță, V.; Anichiti, A.; Brînză, G. The Effectiveness of Online Education during COVID-19 Pandemic—A Comparative Analysis between the Perceptions of Academic Students and High School Students from Romania. *Sustainability* **2021**, *13*, 5311. [CrossRef]
12. Kim, E.-J.; Kim, J.J.; Han, S.-H. Understanding Student Acceptance of Online Learning Systems in Higher Education: Application of Social Psychology Theories with Consideration of User Innovativeness. *Sustainability* **2021**, *13*, 896. [CrossRef]
13. Viner, R.M.; Russell, S.J.; Croker, H.; Packer, J.; Ward, J.; Stansfield, C.; Mytton, O.; Bonell, C.; Booy, R. School closure and management practices during coronavirus outbreaks including COVID-19: A rapid systematic review. *Lancet Child Adolesc. Health* **2020**, *4*, 397–404. [CrossRef]
14. Deogade, S.C.; Naitam, D. COVID-19 and dental aerosols: The infection connection. *Avicenna J. Med.* **2021**, *11*, 107–109. [CrossRef]
15. Epstein, J.B.; Chow, K.; Mathias, R. Dental procedure aerosols and COVID-19. *Lancet Infect. Dis.* **2021**, *21*, e73. [CrossRef]
16. Gambarini, G.; Galli, M.; Gambarini, E.; Di Nardo, D.; Seracchiani, M.; Obino, F.V.; Patil, S.; Bhandi, S.; Miccoli, G.; Testarelli, L. Fine Aerosols and Perceived Risk of COVID-19 among Italian Dental Practitioners: An Experimental Survey. *J. Contemp. Dent. Pract.* **2020**, *21*, 599–603. [CrossRef]
17. Harrel, S.K. Airborne spread of disease—The implications for dentistry. *J. Calif. Dent. Assoc.* **2004**, *32*, 901–906.
18. Harrel, S.K.; Molinari, J. Aerosols and splatter in dentistry: A brief review of the literature and infection control implications. *J. Am. Dent. Assoc.* **2004**, *135*, 429–437. [CrossRef]
19. Forna, N.C. COVID-19 challenges in dental health care and dental schools. *Rom. J. Oral Rehab.* **2020**, *12*, 6–12.
20. CDC, U.; Guidance for Dental Settings. Interim Infection Prevention and Control Guidance for Dental Settings during the COVID-19 Response. Available online: https://www.cdc.gov/coronavirus/2019-ncov/hcp/dental-settings.html (accessed on 20 July 2021).
21. Farooq, I.; Ali, S. COVID-19 outbreak and its monetary implications for dental practices, hospitals and healthcare workers. *Postgrad Med. J.* **2020**, *96*, 791–792. [CrossRef]
22. Ali, S.; Farooq, I.; Abdelsalam, M.; AlHumaid, J. Current Clinical Dental Practice Guidelines and the Financial Impact of COVID-19 on Dental Care Providers. *Eur. J. Dent.* **2020**, *14*, S140–S145. [CrossRef]
23. Machado, R.A.; Bonan, P.R.F.; Perez, D.; Martelli JÚnior, H. COVID-19 pandemic and the impact on dental education: Discussing current and future perspectives. *Braz. Oral Res.* **2020**, *34*, e083. [CrossRef]
24. Chavarría-Bolaños, D.; Gómez-Fernández, A.; Dittel-Jiménez, C.; Montero-Aguilar, M. E-Learning in Dental Schools in the Times of COVID-19: A Review and Analysis of an Educational Resource in Times of the COVID-19 Pandemic. *Odovtos Int. J. Dent. Sci.* **2020**, *22*, 69–86. [CrossRef]
25. Singh, H.K.; Joshi, A.; Malepati, R.N.; Najeeb, S.; Balakrishna, P.; Pannerselvam, N.K.; Singh, Y.K.; Ganne, P. A survey of E-learning methods in nursing and medical education during COVID-19 pandemic in India. *Nurse Educ. Today* **2021**, *99*, 104796. [CrossRef]
26. Parmelee, D.; Michaelsen, L.K.; Cook, S.; Hudes, P.D. Team-based learning: A practical guide: AMEE guide no. 65. *Med. Teach.* **2012**, *34*, e275–e287. [CrossRef]
27. Wang, H.; Xuan, J.; Liu, L.; Shen, X.; Xiong, Y. Problem-based learning and case-based learning in dental education. *Ann. Transl. Med.* **2021**, *9*, 1137. [CrossRef]
28. Jiang, Z.; Zhu, D.; Li, J.; Ren, L.; Pu, R.; Yang, G. Online dental teaching practices during the COVID-19 pandemic: A cross-sectional online survey from China. *BMC Oral Health* **2021**, *21*, 189. [CrossRef]
29. Lewin, K.M. Contingent reflections on coronavirus and priorities for educational planning and development. *Prospects* **2020**, *49*, 17–24. [CrossRef]
30. UMF_Iasi. Available online: https://www.umfiasi.ro/en/academic/facultati/Dental-medicine/Pages/Educational-plans.aspx (accessed on 10 January 2022).
31. Starr, T.N.; Greaney, A.J.; Addetia, A.; Hannon, W.W.; Choudhary, M.C.; Dingens, A.S.; Li, J.Z.; Bloom, J.D. Prospective mapping of viral mutations that escape antibodies used to treat COVID-19. *Science* **2021**, *371*, 850–854. [CrossRef]
32. France, K.; Hangorsky, U.; Wu, C.W.; Sollecito, T.P.; Stoopler, E.T. Participation in an existing massive open online course in dentistry during the COVID-19 pandemic. *J. Dent. Educ.* **2021**, *85*, 78–81. [CrossRef]
33. Iyer, P.; Aziz, K.; Ojcius, D.M. Impact of COVID-19 on dental education in the United States. *J. Dent. Educ.* **2020**, *84*, 718–722. [CrossRef]
34. Schlenz, M.A.; Schmidt, A.; Wöstmann, B.; Krämer, N.; Schulz-Weidner, N. Students' and lecturers' perspective on the implementation of online learning in dental education due to SARS-CoV-2 (COVID-19): A cross-sectional study. *BMC Med. Educ.* **2020**, *20*, 354. [CrossRef]

35. Hattar, S.; AlHadidi, A.; Sawair, F.A.; Alraheam, I.A.; El-Ma'aita, A.; Wahab, F.K. Impact of COVID-19 pandemic on dental education: Online experience and practice expectations among dental students at the University of Jordan. *BMC Med. Educ.* **2021**, *21*, 151. [CrossRef]
36. Varvara, G.; Bernardi, S.; Bianchi, S.; Sinjari, B.; Piattelli, M. Dental Education Challenges during the COVID-19 Pandemic Period in Italy: Undergraduate Student Feedback, Future Perspectives, and the Needs of Teaching Strategies for Professional Development. *Healthcare* **2021**, *9*, 454. [CrossRef]
37. Iurcov, R.; Pop, L.M.; Iorga, M. Impact of COVID-19 Pandemic on Academic Activity and Health Status among Romanian Medical Dentistry Students; A Cross-Sectional Study. *Int. J. Environ. Res. Public Health* **2021**, *18*, 6041. [CrossRef]
38. Goriuc, A.; Sandu, D.; Tatarciuc, M.; Luchian, I. The Impact of the COVID-19 Pandemic on Dentistry and Dental Education: A Narrative Review. *Int. J. Environ. Res. Public Health* **2022**, *19*, 2537. [CrossRef]
39. UMF_Iasi. Serii si Grupe—2020–2021. Available online: https://www.umfiasi.ro/ro/academic/programe-de-studii/licenta/Pagini/Student---Medicin%C4%83-dentar%C4%83.aspx (accessed on 15 February 2022).
40. SurveyMonkey. Available online: https://www.surveymonkey.co.uk/mp/margin-of-error-calculator/ (accessed on 28 August 2022).
41. Deery, C. The COVID-19 pandemic: Implications for dental education. *Evid.-Based Dent.* **2020**, *21*, 46–47. [CrossRef]
42. Fazio, M.; Lombardo, C.; Marino, G.; Marya, A.; Messina, P.; Scardina, G.A.; Tocco, A.; Torregrossa, F.; Valenti, C. LinguAPP: An m-Health Application for Teledentistry Diagnostics. *Int. J. Environ. Res. Public Health* **2022**, *19*, 822. [CrossRef]
43. Elangovan, S.; Mahrous, A.; Marchini, L. Disruptions during a pandemic: Gaps identified and lessons learned. *J. Dent. Educ.* **2020**, *84*, 1270–1274. [CrossRef]
44. Clemente, M.P.; Moreira, A.; Pinto, J.C.; Amarante, J.M.; Mendes, J. The Challenge of Dental Education After COVID-19 Pandemic—Present and Future Innovation Study Design. *Inquiry* **2021**, *58*, 469580211018293. [CrossRef]
45. Goh, P.; Sandars, J. A vision of the use of technology in medical education after the COVID-19 pandemic [version 1]. *MedEdPublish* **2020**, *9*, 49. [CrossRef]
46. Wu, D.T.; Wu, K.Y.; Nguyen, T.T.; Tran, S.D. The impact of COVID-19 on dental education in North America-Where do we go next? *Eur. J. Dent. Educ.* **2020**, *24*, 825–827. [CrossRef]
47. Coughlan, J.; Timuş, D.; Crnic, T.; Srdoč, D.; Halton, C.; Dragan, I.F. Impact of COVID-19 on dental education in Europe: The students' perspective. *Eur. J. Dent. Educ.* **2022**, *26*, 599–607. [CrossRef]
48. Quinn, B.; Field, J.; Gorter, R.; Akota, I.; Manzanares, M.C.; Paganelli, C.; Davies, J.; Dixon, J.; Gabor, G.; Amaral Mendes, R.; et al. COVID-19: The immediate response of european academic dental institutions and future implications for dental education. *Eur. J. Dent. Educ.* **2020**, *24*, 811–814. [CrossRef]
49. Hakami, Z.; Khanagar, S.B.; Vishwanathaiah, S.; Hakami, A.; Bokhari, A.M.; Jabali, A.H.; Alasmari, D.; Aldrees, A.M. Psychological impact of the coronavirus disease 2019 (COVID-19) pandemic on dental students: A nationwide study. *J. Dent. Educ.* **2021**, *85*, 494–503. [CrossRef]
50. Saeed, S.G.; Bain, J.; Khoo, E.; Siqueira, W.L. COVID-19: Finding silver linings for dental education. *J. Dent. Educ.* **2020**, *84*, 1060–1063. [CrossRef] [PubMed]
51. UMF_Iasi. Available online: https://www.umfiasi.ro/ro/Pagini/Suport-psihologic-pentru-comunitatea-UMF-Iasi.aspx (accessed on 28 November 2022).
52. Bennardo, F.; Buffone, C.; Fortunato, L.; Giudice, A. COVID-19 is a challenge for dental education—A commentary. *Eur. J. Dent. Educ.* **2020**, *24*, 822–824. [CrossRef]
53. Li, B.; Cheng, L.; Wang, H. Challenges and Opportunities for Dental Education from COVID-19. *Dent. J.* **2022**, *10*, 188. [CrossRef]
54. Park, J.C.; Kwon, H.E.; Chung, C.W. Innovative digital tools for new trends in teaching and assessment methods in medical and dental education. *J. Educ. Eval. Health Prof.* **2021**, *18*, 13. [CrossRef]
55. Sharab, L.; Adel, M.; Abualsoud, R.; Hall, B.; Albaree, S.; de Leeuw, R.; Kutkut, A. Perception, awareness, and attitude toward digital dentistry among pre-dental students: An observational survey. *Bull. Natl. Res. Cent.* **2022**, *46*, 246. [CrossRef]
56. Meng, L.; Hua, F.; Bian, Z. Coronavirus Disease 2019 (COVID-19): Emerging and Future Challenges for Dental and Oral Medicine. *J. Dent. Res.* **2020**, *99*, 481–487. [CrossRef] [PubMed]
57. Alharbi, F.; Alwadei, S.H.; Alwadei, A.; Asiri, S.; Alwadei, F.; Alqerban, A.; Almuzian, M. Comparison between two asynchronous teaching methods in an undergraduate dental course: A pilot study. *BMC Med. Educ.* **2022**, *22*, 488. [CrossRef]
58. Kunin, M.; Julliard, K.N.; Rodriguez, T.E. Comparing face-to-face, synchronous, and asynchronous learning: Postgraduate dental resident preferences. *J. Dent. Educ.* **2014**, *78*, 856–866. [CrossRef] [PubMed]
59. Kalludi, S.; Punja, D.; Rao, R.; Dhar, M. Is Video Podcast Supplementation as a Learning Aid Beneficial to Dental Students? *J. Clin. Diagn. Res.* **2015**, *9*, Cc04–Cc07. [CrossRef] [PubMed]
60. Prakash, S.S.; Muthuraman, N.; Anand, R. Short-duration podcasts as a supplementary learning tool: Perceptions of medical students and impact on assessment performance. *BMC Med. Educ.* **2017**, *17*, 167. [CrossRef]
61. Zhang, E.; Trad, N.; Corty, R.; Zohrob, D.; Trivedi, S.; Rodman, A. How podcasts teach: A comprehensive analysis of the didactic methods of the top hundred medical podcasts. *Med. Teach.* **2022**, *44*, 1146–1150. [CrossRef] [PubMed]
62. Huang, T.-K.; Yang, C.-H.; Hsieh, Y.-H.; Wang, J.-C.; Hung, C.-C. Augmented reality (AR) and virtual reality (VR) applied in dentistry. *Kaohsiung J. Med. Sci.* **2018**, *34*, 243–248. [CrossRef] [PubMed]

63. Chaturvedi, S.; Elmahdi, A.E.; Abdelmonem, A.M.; Haralur, S.B.; Alqahtani, N.M.; Suleman, G.; Sharif, R.A.; Gurumurthy, V.; Alfarsi, M.A. Predoctoral dental implant education techniques—Students' perception and attitude. *J. Dent. Educ.* **2021**, *85*, 392–400. [CrossRef]
64. Bentata, Y. The COVID-19 pandemic and international federation of medical students' association exchanges: Thousands of students deprived of their clinical and research exchanges. *Med. Educ. Online* **2020**, *25*, 1783784. [CrossRef]
65. Abouzeid, H.; Chaturvedi, S.; Abdelaziz, K.M.; Alzahrani, F.; AlQarni, A.; Alqahtani, N. Role of Robotics and Artificial Intelligence in Oral Health and Preventive Dentistry—Knowledge, Perception and Attitude of Dentists. *Oral Health Prev. Dent.* **2021**, *19*, 353–363. [CrossRef]

International Journal of
Environmental Research and Public Health

MDPI

Article

Certainty in Uncertain Times: Dental Education during the COVID-19 Pandemic–A Qualitative Study

Katja Goetz [1,*], Hans-Jürgen Wenz [2] and Katrin Hertrampf [3]

1 Institute of Family Medicine, University Hospital of Schleswig-Holstein, Campus Lübeck, 23562 Luebeck, Germany
2 Department of Prosthodontics, Propaedeutics and Dental Materials, University Hospital of Schleswig-Holstein, Campus Kiel Germany, 24105 Kiel, Germany
3 Department of Oral and Maxillofacial Surgery, University Hospital of Schleswig-Holstein, Campus Kiel Germany, 24105 Kiel, Germany
* Correspondence: katja.goetz@uni-luebeck.de; Tel.: +49-451-3101-8010

Abstract: Background: The restrictions concerning social contact due to the COVID-19 pandemic implied a rethinking of teaching methods at universities in general, and for practice-oriented teaching such as dental education in particular. This qualitative study aimed to assess aspects of feelings of certainty and uncertainty during this specific education process, incorporating the perspectives of teaching staff and dental students. Methods: Qualitative methods based on interviews were used for data collection. Dental students from different academic years (second, third, fourth, and fifth) and teaching staff responsible for the content and implementation of courses within the dental curriculum were recruited. The data analysis was performed by qualitative content analysis. Results: A total of 39 dental students and 19 teaching staff participated. When students and staff dealt positively with this specific situation, certainty was achieved. The availability of presentations and clear communication enhanced feelings of certainty. The participants often felt unsure about how to handle such a challenging situation and felt insecure when planning for the semester. The students missed contact with other students and argued that the information policy on their dental studies was not transparent enough. In addition, dental students and teaching staff were nervous about the risk of infection from COVID-19, especially in practical courses with patient contact. Conclusions: The COVID-19 pandemic situation leads to a rethinking of dental education. Feelings of certainty can be strengthened by clear and transparent communication as well as training in online teaching methods. To reduce uncertainty, it is crucial to establish channels for information exchange and feedback.

Keywords: COVID-19; dental education; digitalization; practical course; qualitative study; students' experiences; teachers' experiences

Citation: Goetz, K.; Wenz, H.-J.; Hertrampf, K. Certainty in Uncertain Times: Dental Education during the COVID-19 Pandemic–A Qualitative Study. *Int. J. Environ. Res. Public Health* **2023**, *20*, 3090. https://doi.org/10.3390/ijerph20043090

Academic Editor: Giuseppe Alessandro Scardina

Received: 12 January 2023
Revised: 31 January 2023
Accepted: 6 February 2023
Published: 10 February 2023

1. Introduction

In March 2020, COVID-19 was declared by the World Health Organization as a pandemic disease, and this led to severe restrictions on social contact [1]. The social distancing requirements in everyday life also implied a rethinking of teaching methods at universities in general, and for practice-oriented teaching in particular.

Dental education is a very practice-oriented course of study. However, universities worldwide decided to offer a digital summer semester in 2020 to maintain the continuity of dental education [2,3]. As a result, the use of e-learning has significantly expanded. A survey between the end of March and the beginning of April 2020 by the Association of Dental Education in Europe showed that 90% of dental schools used online pedagogical software tools, 72% used live or streamed videos, and 48% provided links to further online materials [4]. However, dental education cannot only be taught digitally. It is a very practical study program. An essential element of the dental curriculum is early and continuous patient contact as part of clinical treatment [5–7]. Students learn competencies that are important for routine treatment processes [8].

Due to the relatively low incidence rates of COVID-19 in Germany's northernmost federal state, senior staff at the Kiel Dental Clinic developed comprehensive social distancing and hygiene measures for the practical courses, and liaised with the relevant local health authority, university, and university hospital. This dental clinic was thus the first clinic in Germany to receive approval under special provision to conduct in-person practical courses with patients from the beginning of May 2020. Theoretical courses were also performed digitally.

Surveys in different countries show that students and clinical staff were relieved that dental education took place digitally. The suspension of face-to-face teaching, especially the practical courses with patients, severely contributed to the loss of students' clinical competence [8–10]. Moreover, different studies show that the new teaching situation negatively impacts the mental health of dental students [11–13]. It is important to know more about how students and teaching staff receive certainty in times of uncertainty for the conceptualization of sustainable training concepts.

Therefore, this study aimed to assess aspects of feelings of certainty and uncertainty during dental education, specifically during the COVID-19 pandemic, at the dental school in Kiel, Germany, by incorporating the perspectives of dental students and their teaching staff.

2. Materials and Methods

2.1. Study Design

This study was designed as a qualitative interview study to assess the experiences of students and teaching staff regarding aspects of certainty and uncertainty, specifically during the COVID-19 pandemic. The consolidated criteria for reporting qualitative research (COREQ) were used [14].

2.2. Participants

Qualitative interviews were conducted with a purposive sample of students and teaching staff. Students from different academic years (second, third, fourth, and fifth) at the dental school in Kiel, Germany, were included in this study, along with associated teaching staff. Dental simulation courses took place in the fourth and sixth semesters, and clinical treatment courses took place from the seventh to tenth semesters. The eighth and tenth semesters were selected as examples for the treatment courses. The target sample consisted of 10 students from each of the four specialist semesters, along with the lecturers from the four departments and the departmental directors (n = 19 in total), taking into account theoretical saturation [15].

For students, the following inclusion criteria were applied: participants of the respective subject per semester, over 18 years of age, and sufficient knowledge of the German language. For lecturers, the inclusion criteria were: responsibility for teaching content and its implementation in one of the Dental Clinic's four departments, over 18 years of age, and sufficient knowledge of the German language. If these criteria were not applied, the participants were excluded from the study.

2.3. Setting

Students were recruited from courses held via video conference in the last third of the summer semester, and lecturers from the various departments were given personal presentations on the project. Participation was voluntary. Appointments for the interviews were then made in person or by email. Data collection took place between June and August 2020. All interviews were conducted by two female members of the working group (K.H.[dental practitioner background], K.G.[health services research background]), either in person or by telephone, and both were experienced in performing qualitative research. As described in the literature, no difference in data quality was observed between face-to-face and telephone interviews, and both may be recommended for use in the same qualitative study [16]. Third persons were not allowed in the interviews. The participants were grouped in such a way that they were unknown to their respective interviewers. All interviews and minuting adhered to the same predefined quality criteria, for example, with documentation of time, field notes, and of any issues or interruptions encountered during the interview. Socio-demographic data was requested from participants before the start of each interview.

2.4. Data Collection

An interdisciplinary team consisting of a sociologist, health services researcher, physician, and dental practitioners developed a semi-structured interview guide. After the final agreement of the guideline by the working group, the two interviewers went through the guideline step by step and agreed on the interview process. This coordination was repeated several times during the interviews. Following a literature review and discussion within the study team, the interview guide (as File S1) focused on two main topics:

- Feelings of certainty due to the experiences of teaching during the COVID-19 pandemic.
- Feelings of uncertainty due to the experiences of teaching during the COVID-19 pandemic.

An identical interview guide was used for both students and teaching staff which was tested with a student and a lecturer. The purpose for the tested interview guide was for comprehensibility and the sequencing of individual questions.

2.5. Data Analysis

All interviews were digitally audio recorded and transcribed in full verbatim. Transcripts were not submitted to participants for comments or correction. The texts were anonymized during transcription before undergoing qualitative content analysis [17]. For data analysis, the software ATLAS.ti 8.4 (Scientific Software Development GmbH, 2020) was used. For the generation of the thematic categories, the research team used a deductive-inductive approach.

Firstly, a provisional category system was developed deductively based on the interview guidelines. Secondly, the provisional category system was then adjusted during analysis according to the content of the transcripts. Any new categories that emerged were then added following an inductive approach. Transcripts were coded independently into the main and subcategories by two female researchers, K.H. (dental practitioner background) and K.G. (health services research background), following intensive discussions that continued until consensus was achieved. Saturation was reached when, during the analyzing process, no new data were added [15]. Participant quotations were translated from German to English for publication purposes. The authors aimed to maintain reflexivity through K.H. and K.G. keeping notes on their thoughts, experiences, reflections, and feelings during the interviews, and discussed how their emotional reactions to participants influenced their interpretation of the results. This study's quality was consistently ensured through adherence to predetermined quality standards. All interviews were conducted by the same two individuals, using the same interview guidelines for all students and teaching staff, under the same conditions. In addition, the proceedings from each interview were documented according to a previously agreed protocol.

2.6. Ethical Approval

This project was approved by the Ethics Committee of the University of Kiel, Germany (D509/20), and was conducted in accordance with the Declaration of Helsinki. Informed consent was obtained via a signed consent form, which included permission to publish anonymized quotes.

3. Results

Overall, 58 interviews were performed—39 with dental students and 19 with teaching staff. Participant characteristics are shown in Table 1 below. The interview duration varied and was about 31 min on average for the dental student group (min. = 22 min, max. = 50 min) and about 31 min for the teaching staff (min. = 15 min, max. = 41 min).

Table 1. Distribution of participants (n = 58).

Variable	Students (n = 39)	Lecturers (n = 19)
Women	27	6
Men	12	13
Age (Mean)	25.2	44.0
(Range of ages)	(20–31)	(31–65)
Apprenticeship	13	-
Further completed study	5	-
Additional qualifications	5	-
Director of the clinic	-	4
Course instructor	-	7
Course assistant	-	8
Use of hardware *:		
Laptop	30	18
Tablet	10	0
Mobile phone	3	0
Stationary PC	2	2
Access to camera (yes)	39	17
Access to microphone (yes)	38	17
Permanent availability	38	17
Adequate internet connection (yes)	38	19
Course in home office		2

* Multiple answers possible.

The following sections describe the two main topics: "Certainty" and "Uncertainty". Quotations are used to illustrate the relevant aspects reported by the participants (students [S] and teaching staff [TS]).

3.1. Main Topic: Certainty

This topic describes what aspects were helpful in creating feelings of certainty in students and teaching staff during the COVID-19 pandemic and the changeover of teaching conditions. For this topic, two main categories were created and divided into different subcategories, as shown in Figure 1 below.

The main category "Own experiences" observed aspects that contributed to the feeling of certainty. It emerged that a certain adjustment to this specific teaching situation was described by both students and teaching staff. Certainty was reached when acclimatization occurred in dealing with this specific situation, especially in applying the tools of online teaching. "I felt comfortable when I got through the first lectures and realized that I could cope well with them and work with them. That's when I started to feel secure" (S36).

Students and teaching staff became experienced in their approach to the situation, as the following statement showed: "But after a time there was routine, so you could also assess whether you felt safe or not" (S14).

The second main category "Stabilizing aspects" comprised different elements that resulted in the feeling of certainty. Clear communication in such a specific situation was perceived as useful: "Everything was communicated clearly, so we were relatively sure how to design the course" (TS06). Students found the support of the teaching staff important for their own feelings of certainty: "Once the semester had been running for two or three weeks, and once you realized that you had the support of the teaching staff" (S04). The supervision of the teaching staff was also ensured during the practical courses under specific regulations, and contributed towards a stabilizing element of certainty: "I would say that I didn't really feel insecure because care was guaranteed. I always had a lecturer who I could call on" (S35). Moreover, students stated that having regular online meetings, such as Zoom meetings with teaching staff, was a helpful aspect of feeling safe.

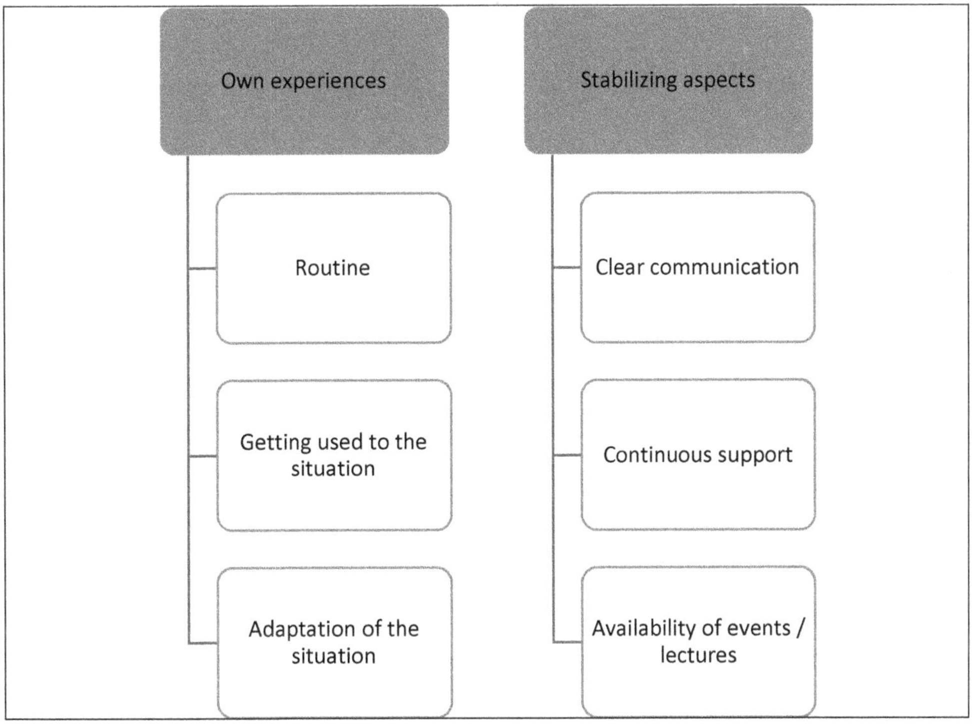

Figure 1. Certainty—main categories and subcategories.

The availability of presentations was another aspect that enhanced certainty: "In terms of the events and the lectures ... I wasn't unsure. I thought to myself: Good, wonderful, I can manage it well" (S22). Students appreciated that the lectures were available on an online platform. Furthermore, the teaching staff also found this an important element for their own certainty: "As I said, I thought that through these online seminars, the students always had the opportunity to listen to the seminars again and again, so to speak, and the lectures again" (TS01). Some of the teaching staff were experienced in dealing with the technical aspects and the implementation of online teaching, and stated that this was important for their own feeling of certainty: "I actually felt relatively sure about the implementation of digitalization, the technical implementation, and the content implementation" (TS02).

3.2. Main Topic: Uncertainty

This topic describes which aspects led to students and teaching staff feeling uncertainty during the COVID-19 pandemic, as well as the change in teaching conditions. Three main categories were created and divided into different subcategories, as shown in Figure 2 below.

The main category "General aspects" comprised statements from the participants regarding how to handle this challenging situation that created general uncertainty during the COVID-19 pandemic, as the following statement from a member of the teaching staff illustrated: "The insecurity I had was due to the uncertainty of the situation. It wasn't one with faulty or improvable behavior, so to speak, but the facts were simply not there and changed every day, and you had to adapt to the changing facts. And that caused the uncertainty" (TS13).

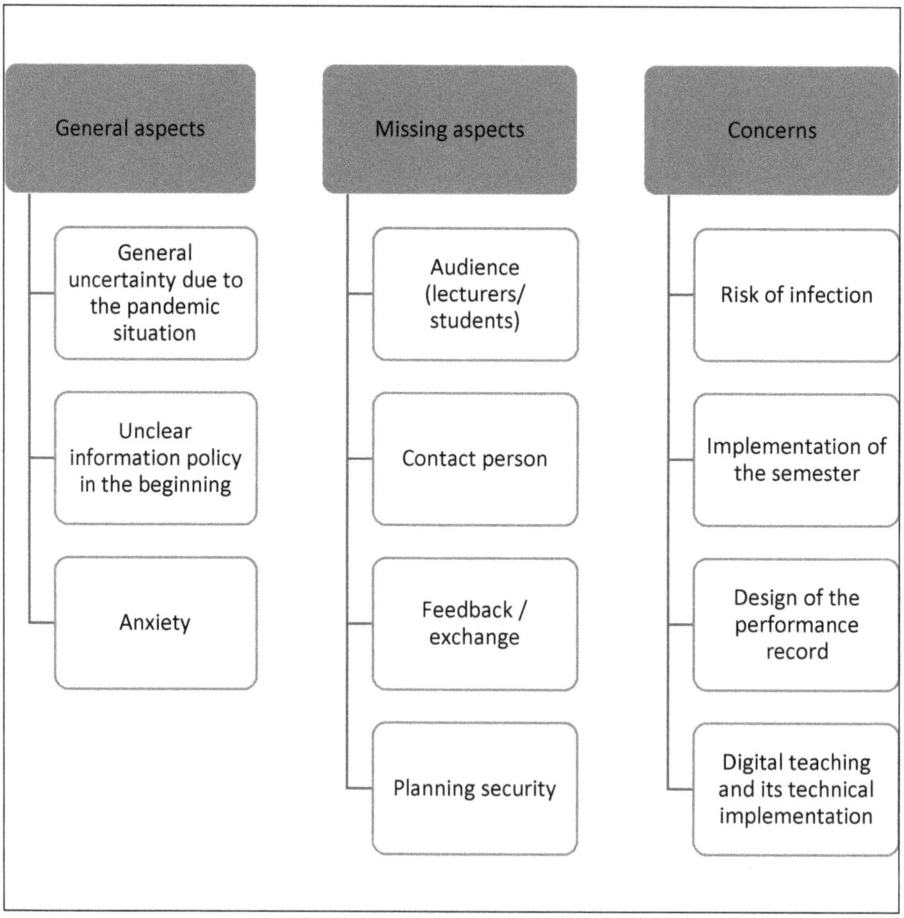

Figure 2. Uncertainty—main categories and subcategories.

Students also felt uncertainty when dealing with such a specific situation: "Uncertainty was there at the beginning, where you didn't know how it would continue, whether it would start, when it would start, how it would proceed" (S01). Furthermore, some students argued that the information policy about their dental studies was not transparent enough: "On the one hand, there was definitely a lack of communication. A lot of information, I think, that was also there, was not communicated to the students or somehow got to them via three corners" (S37). The general perception of the situation, especially the new teaching situation, was often characterized by the term 'anxiety' from students as well as teaching staff. The teaching staff who were responsible for the implementation of the specific regulations and hygienic conditions in the practical courses showed uncertainty concerning implementation and acceptance, as one statement demonstrated: "In the beginning, there was uncertainty in the sense that we were afraid that it wouldn't work. We were afraid that we would fail with the measures we wanted to implement because not everyone would accept them" (TS03).

The main category "Missing aspects" included different issues that both students and teaching staff missed in their daily work. Both groups missed contact with students due to social distancing, and therefore a direct exchange of information or in-person lectures were not possible: "In such an event, where you interact with people in a diminished form, you somehow only have a very brief moment where everyone has the opportunity to ask or say something. I think that gives you a kind of security, when you have the feeling: OK, maybe someone has the same question" (S16).

Nearly all of the teaching staff stated that the change in teaching methods to online-teaching led to a lack of direct feedback during teaching: "What is uncertain and what I don't have is feedback on the extent to which the lecture was received, the extent to which this mediation worked, and how the whole lecture was perceived" (TS02). The lack of knowledge as to whether the content of the lectures reached the students or not was perceived as a feeling of uncertainty by teaching staff: "With these purely digital lectures that you give, I don't feel safe. It's rather ... Well, I don't know if what I'm saying will be received" (TS11).

Some students stated that they missed a direct contact person during the online-teaching: "We felt insecure simply because we didn't have a contact person in that sense" (S26). Due to the situation being unknown, students and teaching staff missed clear planning for the semester. This led to feeling uncertainty.

The teaching staff planned the first lockdown semester with a high level of insecurity, which was accompanied with great uncertainty: "All the planning we did was based on pure thought. We had to adapt to completely new schedules, we had to construct them. And there was a lot of uncertainty as to whether what we were planning for the whole semester was a plan that could be carried out precisely up to the last day. And if it didn't fit, we would have had big problems" (TS13).

The main category of "Concerns" existed during the first lockdown semester, and included the risk of infection, especially in the practical courses, performance during the semester, design of exams, and implementation of online teaching. Students and teaching staff felt uncertain about the risk of being infected with COVID-19, especially in the practical courses with patient contact. "I think with this Corona issue, no one could block it out; certainly no one felt that way. A certain amount of uncertainty always remains, of course, and you also have your patient contacts" (TS11).

Moreover, one member of the teaching staff stated that the patients should to be tested for COVID-19 to provide more certainty: "In the beginning, I think we should have simply tested the patients. That would have given more security" (TS01). Students felt ambivalent about completing the practical course where patients are an integral component, and potentially infectious. "On the one hand, I was thinking: How can I in good conscience call elderly people to come to the clinic? At the time, one simply didn't know how events would develop. And I tell my grandparents: Stay at home. And say to the elderly here: Come to the clinic. That was a bit of an ethical matter, but it was justifiable because we knew that the hygiene concept was right" (S21).

Only some students were concerned as to whether the semester would be completed or not. "I think the biggest uncertainty was whether the semester could take place at all. Digitalization was always just a bit of a side issue. I think the treatment course was central in all our minds" (S02). The majority of students and teaching staff were convinced that the semester would happen. Almost immediately, online tools were implemented for performing online teaching. However, this led to different feelings of uncertainty from the students and teaching staff. One member of the teaching staff stated: "Yes, it is different. The uncertainty was related to the way how I record the presentation or put it online practically, whether I'm not overwhelming the students with it or demanding more" (TS08).

Students were not sure about what kind of content could be provided within dental studies: "Yes, I think in the beginning there was uncertainty as to whether all the content could really be conveyed digitally, whether you would really get to grips with every topic in that sense" (S14). The technical implementation and use of different tools and devices were a challenge for some participants. "The first few times I logged into Zoom events, I sometimes didn't know if it was the right thing to do, or if I had to click on it, or if I was going to miss it" (S11).

4. Discussion

The results show that different aspects could influence feelings of certainty and uncertainty during such a specific education process during the COVID-19 pandemic. The perspectives of dental students and their teaching staff are considered, and the various statements show that a process from uncertainty to certainty could be observed. As our results demonstrate, clear communication led to feelings of certainty and was also found in other studies [9]. However, the unclear information policy at the beginning of the online teaching situation and the practical courses under specific regulations was due to the situation itself. Never before have people experienced such a pandemic; they could not anticipate the consequences.

Different studies with dental students and their educators show the challenges during dental education and their effect on clinical performance [9,10,18]. In most countries, dental education changed to online education, which was perceived positively by dental students [4,18]. On the one hand, social distancing in terms of online teaching could minimize the infection rate of COVID-19 and lead to a feeling of certainty. On the other hand, social distancing could lead to the loss of a supportive network and create stress for students. Social support, such as by teaching staff, was found to be an important stabilizing element and was also observed as a protective factor concerning emotional loneliness [19,20].

Face-to-face exchanges and communication allow people to read non-verbal signals, but with social distancing, these non-verbal signals are absent, which could lead to a difficult communication process. The direct feedback that helps to assess whether a peer understands the meaning of the statement could lead to a sense of uncertainty in the communication process. Furthermore, it was found that the lack of peer feedback could have a negative impact on the effectiveness of online learning [21]. It can be assumed that the uncertainties over the outcome of the pandemic could have an effect on teaching staff as well as students' well-being.

As already mentioned, the practical courses with patients started at the beginning of May 2020 with the concept of rigorous hygiene. However, this was associated with two main concerns: fear of infection, and completing the practical courses during the semester. Both concerns led to feelings of uncertainty for students and the teaching staff. Different studies show that the risk of COVID-19 infection was one of the reasons to perform any kind of education digitally [9,10,22,23]. From our perspective, we have not seen any students or teaching staff infected by COVID-19 within the practical courses during the first COVID-19 semester. Uncertainty has been replaced by a sense of security. Moreover, sustainable training concepts such as the field of technical competencies and the strengthening of mental health are necessary to become resilient in uncertain times.

Limitations

This study has several limitations. The results cannot be generalized without further research because of the design of the qualitative study. Self-reporting comments from the students and teaching staff were used to present the results of this qualitative study. It is therefore not possible to make any assessments about the accuracy of the information. Moreover, participation in the interviews was voluntary. It must also be assumed that the study attracted interested students and teaching staff who were more open to the topics discussed. This "positive selection bias" may be reflected in the results and thus needs to be taken into account during interpretation.

5. Conclusions

The COVID-19 pandemic situation is a challenge for dental education, especially for the practical courses. Different aspects seem important for a sense of certainty and should be considered for future teaching situations. Clear and transparent communication would be useful, as well as training in online teaching methods, to strengthen the feeling of certainty. To reduce uncertainty in a pandemic situation, it is particularly important to establish channels for communication, information exchange, and feedback. In addition, this study provides empirical evidence and insight into the aspects that lead to feelings of certainty and uncertainty by dental students and their teaching staff during the COVID-19 crisis.

Supplementary Materials: The following supporting information can be downloaded at: https://www.mdpi.com/article/10.3390/ijerph20043090/s1, File S1: Interview guide for lectures and students.

Author Contributions: K.G.: conceptualization, methodology, investigation, formal analysis, and writing—original draft; H.-J.W.: conceptualization, methodology, and writing—review; K.H.: conceptualization, methodology, resources, project administration, investigation, formal analysis, and writing—original draft. All authors have read and agreed to the published version of the manuscript.

Funding: This study was supported by the Medical Faculty of the Christian-Albrechts-University, Kiel.

Institutional Review Board Statement: This project was approved by the Ethics Committee of the University of Kiel, Germany (D509/20), and was conducted in accordance with the Declaration of Helsinki. Informed consent was obtained via a signed consent form, which included permission to publish anonymized quotes.

Informed Consent Statement: Informed consent was obtained from all subjects involved in the study and written informed consent has been obtained from the participants to publish this paper.

Data Availability Statement: The datasets generated during the current study are not publicly available due to the ethical requirements, but are available from the corresponding author upon reasonable request.

Acknowledgments: We would like to acknowledge and thank all participants for their contribution and insight.

Conflicts of Interest: The authors declare no conflict of interest.

References

1. Mahase, E. China coronavirus: WHO declares international emergency as death toll exceeds 200. *BMJ* **2020**, *368*, m408. [CrossRef] [PubMed]
2. Chang, T.Y.; Hong, G.; Paganelli, C.; Phantumvanit, P.; Chang, W.J.; Shieh, Y.S.; Hsu, M.L. Innovation of dental education during COVID-19 pandemic. *J. Dent. Sci.* **2021**, *16*, 15–20. [CrossRef] [PubMed]
3. Iyer, P.; Aziz, K.; Ojcius, D.M. Impact of COVID-19 on dental education in the United States. *J. Dent. Educ.* **2020**, *84*, 718–722. [CrossRef] [PubMed]
4. Quinn, B.; Field, J.; Gorter, R.; Akota, I.; Manzanares, M.C.; Paganelli, C.; Davies, J.; Dixon, J.; Gabor, G.; Amaral Mendes, R.; et al. COVID-19: The immediate response of European academic dental institutions and future implications for dental education. *Eur. J. Dent. Educ.* **2020**, *24*, 811–814. [CrossRef]
5. Hattar, S.; AlHadidi, A.; Sawair, F.A.; Alraheam, I.A.; El-Ma'aita, A.; Wahab, F.K. Impact of COVID-19 pandemic on dental education: Online experience and practice expectations among dental students at the University of Jordan. *BMC Med. Educ.* **2021**, *21*, 151–160. [CrossRef]
6. Nasseripour, M.; Turner, J.; Rajadurai, S.; San Diego, J.; Quinn, B.; Bartlett, A.; Volponi, A.A. COVID 19 and dental education: Transitioning from a well-established synchronous format and face to face teaching to an asynchronous format of dental clinical teaching and learning. *J. Med. Educ. Curric. Dev.* **2021**, *8*, 2382120521999667. [CrossRef]
7. Varvara, G.; Bernardi, S.; Bianchi, S.; Sinjari, B.; Piattelli, M. Dental education challenges during the COVID-19 pandemic period in Italy: Undergraduate student feedback, future perspectives, and the needs of teaching strategies for professional development. *Healthcare* **2021**, *9*, 454. [CrossRef]
8. Jum'ah, A.A.; Elsalem, L.; Loch, C.; Schwass, D.; Brunton, P.A. Perception of health and educational risks amongst dental students and educators in the era of COVID-19. *Eur. J. Dent. Educ.* **2021**, *25*, 506–515. [CrossRef]
9. Hung, M.; Licari, F.W.; Hon, E.S.; Lauren, E.; Su, S.; Birmingham, W.C.; Wadsworth, L.L.; Lassetter, J.H.; Graff, T.C.; Harman, W.; et al. In an era of uncertainty: Impact of COVID-19 on dental education. *J. Dent. Educ.* **2021**, *85*, 148–156. [CrossRef]
10. Loch, C.; Kuan, I.B.J.; Elsalem, L.; Schwass, D.; Brunton, P.A.; Jum'ah, A. COVID-19 and dental clinical practice: Students and clinical staff perceptions of health risks and educational impact. *J. Dent. Educ.* **2021**, *85*, 44–52. [CrossRef]
11. Hakami, Z.; Vishwanathaiah, S.; Abuzinadah, S.H.; Alhaddad, A.J.; Bokhari, A.M.; Marghalani, H.Y.A.; Shahin, S.Y. Effects of COVID-19 lockdown on the mental health of dental students: A longitudinal study. *J. Dent. Educ.* **2021**, *85*, 1854–1862. [CrossRef]
12. Agius, A.M.; Gatt, G.; Vento Zahra, E.; Busuttil, A.; Gainza-Cirauqui, M.L.; Cortes, A.R.G.; Attard, N.J. Self-reported dental student stressors and experiences during the COVID-19 pandemic. *J. Dent. Educ.* **2021**, *85*, 208–215. [CrossRef]
13. Etajuri, E.A.; Mohd, N.R.; Naimie, Z.; Ahmad, N.A. Undergraduate dental students' perspective of online learning and their physical and mental health during COVID-19 pandemic. *PLoS ONE* **2022**, *17*, e0270091. [CrossRef]

14. Tong, A.; Sainsbury, P.; Craig, J. Consolidated criteria for reporting qualitative research (COREQ): A 32-item checklist for interviews and focus groups. *Int. J. Qual. Health Care* **2007**, *19*, 349–357. [CrossRef]
15. Bowen, G.A. Naturalistic inquiry and the saturation concept: A research note. *Qual. Res.* **2008**, *8*, 137–152. [CrossRef]
16. Sturges, J.E.; Hanrahan, K.J. Comparing telephone and face-to-face qualitative interviewing: A research note. *Qual. Res.* **2004**, *4*, 107–118. [CrossRef]
17. Mayring, P. *Qualitative Inhaltsanalyse*, 11th ed.; Beltz: Weinheim, Germany, 2010.
18. Machado, A.R.; Bonan, P.R.F.; Perez, D.E.C.; Martelli Júnior, H. COVID-19 pandemic and the impact on dental education: Discussing current and future perspectives. *Braz. Oral Res.* **2020**, *34*, e083. [CrossRef]
19. Labrague, L.J.; de los Santos, J.A.A.; Falguera, C.C. Social and emotional loneliness among college students during the COVID-19 pandemic: The predictive role of coping behaviors, social support, and personal resilience. *Perspect. Psychiatr. Care* **2021**, *57*, 1578–1584. [CrossRef]
20. Guse, J.; Weegen, A.S.; Heinen, I.; Bergelt, C. Mental burden and perception of the study situation among undergraduate students during the COVID-19 pandemic: A cross-sectional study and comparison of dental and medical students. *BMJ Open* **2021**, *11*, e054728. [CrossRef]
21. Kara, N. Enablers and barriers of online-learning during the COVID-19 pandemic: A case study of an online university course. *J. Univ. Teach. Learn. Pract.* **2021**, *18*, 130–146. [CrossRef]
22. Ihm, L.; Zhang, H.; van Vijfeijken, A.; Waugh, M.G. Impacts of the COVID-19 pandemic on the health of university students. *Int. J. Health Plan. Manag.* **2021**, *36*, 618–627. [CrossRef] [PubMed]
23. Procentese, F.; Esposito, C.; Gonzalez Leone, F.; Agueli, B.; Arcidiacono, C.; Freda, M.F.; Di Napoli, I. Psychological lockdown experiences: Downtime or an unexpected time for being? *Front. Psychol.* **2021**, *12*, 577089. [CrossRef] [PubMed]

International Journal of
Environmental Research and Public Health

MDPI

Article

Filter Masks during the Second Phase of SARS-CoV-2: Study on Population

Enzo Cumbo, Giuseppe Gallina, Pietro Messina and Giuseppe Alessandro Scardina *

Department of Surgical Oncological and Stomatological Disciplines, University of Palermo, Via Del Vespro 129, 90127 Palermo, Italy
* Correspondence: alessandro.scardina@unipa.it

Abstract: During the SARS-CoV-2 pandemic, the most common countermeasure are the use of masks, which are supposed to filter inhaled and exhaled air to reduce the spread of the virus. The masks, which are medical devices, must be used by providing appropriate instructions for correct use. This study, which examined the population during the advanced stage of the pandemic, highlighted a substantial improvement in the management and choice of masks, even though the information disseminated to the population probably should be even more detailed and precise in order to avoid incorrect behavior that could compromise the effectiveness of these devices; in fact a high percentage of subjects had behaviors that can facilitate the spread of the virus, such as the continuous attempts to correct the incorrect positioning of the mask on the face or the need to move it because it is annoying.

Keywords: COVID-19; masks; information; incorrect behavior

Citation: Cumbo, E.; Gallina, G.; Messina, P.; Scardina, G.A. Filter Masks during the Second Phase of SARS-CoV-2: Study on Population. *Int. J. Environ. Res. Public Health* **2023**, *20*, 2360. https://doi.org/10.3390/ijerph20032360

Academic Editor: Fawad Javed

Received: 2 December 2022
Revised: 26 January 2023
Accepted: 27 January 2023
Published: 29 January 2023

1. Introduction

The COVID-19 pandemic is nowadays a fairly well-known and studied disease for which it is understood that it is necessary to limit the airborne spread of this virus in every way.

One of the solutions most adopted by governments was the lockdown, through which the citizens of most nations were forced to stay inside their homes for months, completely canceling all social relations. Another countermeasure was that of "social distancing", which literally prevented non-cohabiting subjects, when they were outside their homes, from staying close to each other, thus avoiding the gatherings that would facilitate the infections. Mass vaccination further helped the fight against COVID-19 and strengthened our immune defenses against this microorganism to which we had no immunity whatsoever. Other concepts, of which attempts were made in all countries to disseminate information, are concepts relating to personal hygiene, and above all, hygiene of the hands, by numerous advising commercials and demonstration videos; to this was also added the ubiquitous availability of disinfectant gels present in most places accessible to the public, such as stores. Finally, the imposition of the use of filter masks by governments of most of the entire planet represented another fundamental decision with the intention of limiting the circulation of the virus as much as possible, especially when citizens were confined in spaces that were poorly ventilated [1–4].

The massive use of filter masks, in normal daily activities, helped to contain the contagion among the population because the transmission of this virus occurs mainly by air [5–9].

However, we must consider the way in which the mask is managed by people who, when the pandemic began to spread, were not adequately informed on how to behave [10,11].

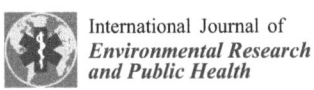

That lack of precise information certainly led the population to make serious mistakes using those masks; they were often worn of not covering their nose and mouth correctly. All this led to a reduction in the filtering efficiency of this device, reducing its effectiveness

in a historical moment when the lack of mass vaccination prompted doctors to try to reduce the airborne spread of the virus by any means [12,13].

Most likely, the breathing difficulties caused by this filter led the population not to wear it correctly; in fact, the FFP2, and above all, the FFP3 masks, were little used at the beginning of the pandemic precisely because they made breathing difficult, and also due to their shape, which is made to make the edges adhere well to the face. These difficulties, together with the fact that the population was not at all used to circulating wearing such medical devices, often led citizens to leave the mask itself non-adherent to the skin, letting unfiltered air pass both during inspiration and expiration, invalidating its function.

In addition, people who are particularly intolerant of the breathing difficulties caused by filtering masks chose to wear those with valves that filter only the inhaled air, leaving the exhaled air, which could be potentially infected, to escape unfiltered.

To this is added an incorrect management, such as touching the mask repeatedly because it is a source of discomfort or trying to position it better on the face. These incorrect behaviors can make the masks even more ineffective or make them a dangerous vehicle for the spread of the disease itself.

Nowadays, in order to drastically reduce the problems mentioned, a massive information campaign was organized in all countries, which tried to spread the correct use of this important medical device.

However, it is important to underline that all governments, during the first phase of the pandemic, focused their attention on simply advising the use of masks, and only when the infection began to show its danger and uncontrollability did they resort to the formulation of laws, which more or less rigidly imposed the use of this device. Initially, there were no particular indications on the type of mask to wear and any type was fine, but when awareness of the extent of the problem increased, governments focused not only on the quantity, but also on the quality of filtering devices, directing the population towards models with better performance, such as FFP2/FFP3.

As the months went by, the dissemination of information on how to wear these devices in order to optimize their filtering effect became increasingly important.

During this second phase, it is less frequent to witness incorrect behaviors that nullify or drastically reduce the filtering power of the masks.

This study aims to verify if, during this advanced phase of the COVID-19 pandemic, the population changed the way they use and manage filter masks, given that the information on their use is widely spread worldwide [14–17].

During the use of masks, in addition to considering the way in which they are worn, it is also essential to focus attention on daily management.

As with all filtering devices, even masks can easily become infected, paradoxically becoming a vehicle for virus transmission. The risk of spreading the microorganisms trapped on the surface of this filter is linked, for example, to the continuous touching or adjusting the position of the mask itself; this leads to an unaware contamination of the hands with which other objects or surfaces are touched, which in turn become infected. For this reason, this research also investigated this important aspect, which is just as important as wearing the mask correctly [18].

2. Material and Method

This research was conducted in Italy (March 2022) and investigated the way in which the mask was worn and managed by the population.

The observation of the sample was carried out in large commercial establishments where the need to wear filter masks was particularly felt by people because the probability of contracting the infection is certainly greater in closed and crowded places.

Particular attention was paid to go unnoticed during the observation period so as not to influence, in any case, the behavior of the subjects in the sample.

In this way all the observed people acted in an absolutely natural way, unaware of being watched.

The research was conducted over a 15-day period from 9:00 A.M. to 08:00 P.M.; in the choice of the representative sample, children were deliberately excluded because their "non-rational behavior" could distort the result.

The number of subjects examined was 1084; the observation time for each individual subject was 60 s.

This study looked at various parameters, such as type of mask (surgical mask, FFP2/FFP3 with valve, FFP2/FFP3 without valve, and self-made or cloth-replaced mask), correct wearing (covering nose, mouth, and chin), and the correct management (touching or not the mask on the external surface).

All data were collected by a single observer who, placed at a distance of about 5 m from the subject under observation, used pre-compiled forms, inserted into a smart phone, in which several fields were present. Each observed subject was assigned a sequential numerical code, which guaranteed anonymity; moreover, no photographs were ever taken in order to respect privacy. In each single module, the possible scenarios were already indicated, such as the various types of masks worn or if it was positioned correctly on the face and/or touched with the hands.

In this way, the observer only had to place a flag on the form; this facilitated both the collection of data and the fact that whoever collected them went completely unnoticed.

In order to make the presence of the observer even more discreet, the latter after the observation period, equal to sixty seconds, moved to a distance in another area or another floor of the store, in order not to arouse suspects and undertake undisturbed observation on another research sample.

All collected data were statistically analyzed by chi-square test.

3. Results

The observation of 1084 subjects in commercial activities showed that a large number of people wore filter masks (97.98%) and only a very small part of the sample (2.02%) did not protect their nose and mouth regardless of the danger of spreading the virus by air.

Among the subjects wearing masks, the preference was towards the FFP2/FFP3 type without a valve (93.72%), followed by the surgical type, even if only noticed on a fairly small number of people (2.95%). Even lower was the number of subjects who wore an FFP2/FFP3 with a valve (1.10%), and only a couple of people (0.18%) tried to self-build a protective mask.

As regards the ways in which the filter masks were worn by the sample, the following results are highlighted:

Among the subjects who wore surgical masks, it was found that many of them did it correctly (75%); only a few people (25%) made mistakes by not covering the nose, mouth, or chin, or leaving the mask loose on the face, thus reducing the filtering capacity.

People who wore FFP2/FFP3 masks without valves showed that they did it correctly in most cases (92.32%), and only a small number of subjects observed with this type of mask did not adequately cover their nose, mouth, and chin (7.67%).

The research also revealed that most of the people with FFP2/FFP3 masks with a valve wore the medical device appropriately (83.33%) and only a few subjects did not wear it correctly (16.66%).

Only two people were noticed with self-made masks and in both cases the "devices" were worn incorrectly (100%) (Table 1).

Table 1. Distribution of result about wearing.

Correctness in Wearing	No Mask n (%)	Surgical Mask n (%)	FFP2/FFP3 No Valve n (%)	FFP2/FFP3 with Valve n (%)	Self Made Mask n (%)
	22 (2.02%)	**32 (2.95%)**	**1016 (93.72%)**	**12 (1.10%)**	**2 (0.18%)**
Correct	not applicable	24 (75%)	938 (92.32%)	10 (83.33%)	0 (0%)
Incorrect	not applicable	8 (25%)	78 (7.67%)	2 (16.66%)	2 (100%)

The study also reported data on the subjects' behavior towards worn filtering devices and the results are as follows:

Among the people who wore surgical masks, about half (53.12%) did not touch the medical device during the observation period; the other subjects (46.87%) did it at least once, and some of them repeatedly.

Even considering the people who wore FFP2/FFP3 without a valve, more than half of them (57.66%) did not touch the mask during the observation period, but a still large number of the sample (42.31%) did it once or more times.

The very few people who wore FFP2/FFP3 with a valve showed (58.33%) that they did not touch the mask, but a large number of them (41.66%) still touched the device with their hands.

Only two people wore self-made masks and both (100%) touched them even more times (Table 2).

Table 2. Distribution of result about management.

Management	No Mask n (%)	Surgical Mask n (%)	FFP2/FFP3 No Valve n (%)	FFP2/FFP3 with Valve n (%)	Self Made Mask n (%)
	22 (2.02%)	**32 (2.95%)**	**1016 (93.72%)**	**12 (1.10%)**	**2 (0.18%)**
Good management	not applicable	17 (53.12%)	586 (57.66%)	7 (58.3%)	0 (0%)
Bad managment	not applicable	15 (46.87%)	430 (42.31%)	5 (41.6%)	2 (100%)

4. Discussion

The filter masks, which are widely used in medicine and in all those fields in which it is necessary to filter the inhaled and exhaled air, represent an excellent means of containing the spread of microbes that spread through the air.

All medical devices must be accompanied by precise instructions on use and maintenance in order to fully exploit their potential. In this particular historical moment, where a medical device was imposed on the population, it emerged that informing is as important as imposing.

Our study showed that any type of filter mask must be worn and managed very carefully; otherwise, it completely loses its effectiveness [19–21].

At the beginning of when the COVID-19 pandemic started, the population was certainly not prepared to properly use a device that is normally intended for health personnel [22,23].

This happened because when governments began to spread information on masks, they could not imagine how much such a seemingly simple-to-use device needed detailed information on how to use it, what to do, and also what not to do in order to prevent a filter mask, which has the task of preventing infections, from turning into a vehicle of contagion instead.

During the pandemic months, the compounding information played a decisive role in improving the management of these masks that seem of trivial usefulness, but which hide various criticalities and problems.

It is important to note that, during the second phase of the pandemic, the percentage of the sample who did not wear filter masks was really low (2.02%); this low percentage shows that the perception of the pandemic problem is very different from the initial period when general disorientation and misinformation prevailed. In fact, in the first months of the pandemic, a large part of the population was particularly skeptical even about the real existence of the infection, and in any case, the use of masks was sporadic [24].

The very low percentage of subjects observed with self-made masks (0.18%) confirms the greater diffusion of information among the population that basically understood that they cannot self-build a medical device, putting their own health and that of others at risk. At the beginning of the pandemic, in attempts to self-build masks, the population showed the greatest inspiration, but with particularly poor medical results; often, pieces of cloth with undoubted filtering capacity were simply used, literally placed on the face or tied in an approximate way or held in place with the hands in a discontinuous manner. This was the most striking demonstration of disinformation shown by the population [25,26].

Differently from our previous study, where the surgical masks were the most observed, in this new research, the data changed, and the most encountered masks were the FFP2/FFP3 without valves (93.72%), which represent the type suggested and/or imposed by the majority of European nations. This means that, for the same number of subjects wearing filter masks, a very high percentage of subjects with FFP2/FFP3 are much less likely to spread the virus [27].

Touching an infected mask with your hands could facilitate the contamination of other objects; all of this could happen, for example, with an infected and asymptomatic patient who, unaware of being infected with COVID-19, while correctly wearing a type of mask with a high filtering power such as FFP3, due to the breathing difficulties it could cause, repeatedly touches the device infecting his hands, which in turn become a means of spreading the virus [28,29].

As confirmation of how confused and imprecise the diffusion of the concepts of microbiology are in the population, it is interesting to note how almost all of the customers, observed inside the commercial shops, used the sanitizing gel provided at the entrance to reduce the microbial load on their hands; unfortunately the same subjects then repeatedly touched their potentially infected masks, probably unaware of having made useless the use of the disinfectant gel used a few minutes before [30].

All governments, in addition to giving indications on the type of mask to wear and how to use it correctly, probably should accompany their information with teachings of microbiology concepts that are easily accessible to the entire population.

This is not easy to do, because the level of basic biological knowledge can be very variable within the population, which is very uneven in all countries. These years of pandemic, therefore, put a strain on all the nations that tried, in various ways, to inform citizens in the best way, even if the strategic choices adopted and the information given to citizens did not always prove successful; to this is added that often within the same nation, the information released over time was discordant and misleading, therefore also losing credibility. The various strategic decisions, given by the various nations on the guidelines for citizens, also contributed to aggravating the disorientation [31].

5. Conclusions

The main enemy of this pandemic is an invisible microorganism; and the data in our possession confirm that it is particularly difficult to spread microbiological and medical information on infections to the "non-medical" population who are not used to fighting microscopic, and above all, invisible viruses capable of contaminating the air we breathe and the surfaces of the objects we live with on a daily basis.

This explains why even the people most attentive to wearing masks correctly that observed in our research often touched them without considering that these devices could potentially be infected, and therefore become a vehicle for transmission.

However, the study highlights how these years of pandemic made the population understand the importance of wearing proper masks, especially in closed and crowded places where the probability of spreading the virus is greater.

The high percentage of subjects identified as wearing FFP2/FFP3 masks confirms that choices on the type of mask to wear are also made on the basis of information widely disseminated by governments.

However, the data on the correct use of masks, which emerged from this study, indicate that the population needs some more information on how to manage this medical device.

The imposition of these masks and the dissemination by the government of correct information on how to wear them is a winning factor in the attempt to reduce the spread of the COVID-19 virus; but on the occasion of extraordinary events, such as the SARS-CoV-2 pandemic, information messages must be particularly clear, targeted, and repetitive without neglecting any aspect in order to reduce behavioral errors in the population.

It should be emphasized that our research, while revealing a high percentage of subjects wearing appropriate filtering masks, shows that poor management of masks is still widespread in the population; in fact, both attempts to correct the wrong positioning of the device on the face and the need to move it continuously because it is annoying are still too frequent.

The key words, in situations such as those that the pandemic imposed on the entire planet, seem to be clarity and dissemination of certain information supported by scientific evidence in order to avoid useless and harmful misunderstandings in the population.

Author Contributions: Methodology, E.C.; Validation, G.G. and P.M.; Investigation, G.A.S. All authors have read and agreed to the published version of the manuscript.

Funding: This research received no external funding.

Institutional Review Board Statement: Ethical review and approval were waived for this study because this is an observational research on population without any involvement. The study was conducted in accordance with the Declaration of Helsinki.

Informed Consent Statement: Not applicable.

Data Availability Statement: Data supporting reported results can be asked to enzo.cumbo@unipa.it.

Conflicts of Interest: The authors declare no conflict of interest.

References

1. Lai, C.C.; Shih, T.P.; Ko, W.C.; Tang, H.J.; Hsueh, P.R. Severe acute respiratory syndrome coronavirus 2 (SARS-CoV-2) and coronavirus disease-2019 (COVID-19): The epidemic and the challenges. *Int. J. Antimicrob. Agents* **2020**, *55*, 105924. [CrossRef] [PubMed]
2. Gumel, A.B.; Ruan, S.; Day, T.; Watmough, J.; Brauer, F.; Driessche, P.V.D.; Gabrielson, D.; Bowman, C.; Alexander, M.E.; Ardal, S.; et al. Modelling strategies for controlling SARS outbreaks. *Proc. Biol. Sci.* **2004**, *271*, 2223–2232. [CrossRef] [PubMed]
3. Zhang, R.; Li, Y.; Zhang, A.L.; Wang, Y.; Molina, M.J. Identifying airborne transmission as the dominant route for the spread of COVID-19. *Proc. Natl. Acad. Sci. USA* **2020**, *26*, 14857–14863. [CrossRef] [PubMed]
4. Leung, N.H.L.; Chu, D.K.W.; Shiu, E.Y.C.; Chan, K.-H.; McDevitt, J.J.; Hau, B.J.P.; Yen, H.-L.; Li, Y.; Ip, D.K.M.; Peiris, J.S.M.; et al. Respiratory virus shedding in exhaled breath and efficacy of face masks. *Nat. Med.* **2020**, *26*, 676–680. [CrossRef]
5. MacIntyre, C.R.; Chughtai, A.A. Facemasks for the prevention of infection in healthcare and community settings. *BMJ* **2015**, *350*, 694. [CrossRef] [PubMed]
6. Lipp, A. The effectiveness of surgical face masks: What the literature shows. *Nurs. Times* **2003**, *99*, 22–24.
7. Coclite, D.; Napoletano, A.; Gianola, S.; Del Monaco, A.; D'Angelo, D.; Fauci, A.; Iacorossi, L.; Latina, R.; Torre, G.L.; Mastroianni, C.M.; et al. Face mask use in the community for reducing the spread of COVID-19: A systematic review. *Front. Med.* **2021**, *7*, 594269. [CrossRef]

8. Eikenberry, S.E.; Mancuso, M.; Iboi, E.; Phan, T.; Eikenberry, K.; Kuang, Y.; Kostelich, E.; Gumel, A.B. To mask or not to mask: Modeling the potential for face mask use by the general public to curtail the COVID-19 pandemic. *Infect. Dis. Model.* **2020**, *5*, 293–308. [CrossRef]
9. Ueki, H.; Furusawa, Y.; Iwatsuki-Horimoto, K.; Imai, M.; Kabata, H.; Nishimura, H.; Kawaoka, Y. Effectiveness of face masks in preventing airborne transmission of SARS-CoV-2. *MSphere* **2020**, *5*, e00637-20. [CrossRef] [PubMed]
10. MacIntyre, C.R.; Cauchemez, S.; Dwyer, D.E.; Seale, H.; Cheung, P.; Browne, G.; Fasher, M.; Wood, J.; Gao, Z.; Booy, R.; et al. Face mask use and control of respiratory virus transmission in households. *Emerg. Infect. Dis.* **2010**, *15*, 233. [CrossRef]
11. Jefferson, T.; Foxlee, R.; Del Mar, C.; Dooley, L.; Ferroni, E.; Hewak, B.; Prabhala, A.; Nair, S.; Rivetti, A. Physical interventions to interrupt or reduce the spread of respiratory viruses: Systematic review. *Br. Med. J.* **2008**, *336*, 77–80. [CrossRef]
12. Gibney, E. Whose coronavirus strategy worked best? Scientists hunt most effective policies. *Nature* **2020**, *581*, 15–16. [CrossRef] [PubMed]
13. Nakayachi, K.; Ozaki, T.; Shibata, Y.; Yokoi, R. Why do Japanese people use masks against COVID-19, even though masks are unlikely to offer protection from infection? *Front. Psychol.* **2020**, *11*, 1918. [CrossRef] [PubMed]
14. Betsch, C.; Korn, L.; Sprengholz, P.; Felgendreff, L.; Eitze, S.; Schmid, P.; Böhm, R. Social and behavioral consequences of mask policies during the COVID-19 pandemic. *Proc. Natl. Acad. Sci. USA* **2020**, *117*, 21851–21853. [CrossRef] [PubMed]
15. Chung, J.B.; Kim, B.J.; Kim, E.S. Mask-wearing behavior during the COVID-19 pandemic in Korea: The role of individualism in a collectivistic country. *Int. J. Disaster Risk Reduct.* **2022**, *82*, 103355. [CrossRef] [PubMed]
16. Bir, C.; Widmar, N.O. Societal values and mask usage for COVID-19 control in the US. *Prev. Med.* **2021**, *153*, 106784. [CrossRef]
17. Tso, R.V.; Cowling, B.J. Importance of face masks for COVID-19: A call for effective public education. *Clin. Infect. Dis.* **2020**, *71*, 2195–2198. [CrossRef]
18. Prather, K.A.; Wang, C.C.; Schooley, R.T. Reducing transmission of SARS-CoV-2. *Science* **2020**, *368*, 1422–1424. [CrossRef]
19. Bałazy, A.; Toivola, M.; Adhikari, A.; Sivasubramani, S.K.; Reponen, T.; Grinshpun, S.A. Do N95 Respirators Provide 95% Protection Level Against Airborne Viruses, and How Adequate Are Surgical Masks? *Am. J. Infect. Control* **2006**, *34*, 51–57. [CrossRef]
20. Chen, C.C.; Willeke, K. Characteristics of face seal leakage in filtering facepieces. *Am. Ind. Hyg. Assoc. J.* **1992**, *53*, 533–539. [CrossRef]
21. MacIntyre, C.R.; Chughtai, A.A. A rapid systematic review of the efficacy of face masks and respirators against coronaviruses and other respiratory transmissible viruses for the community, healthcare workers and sick patients. *Int. J. Nurs. Stud.* **2020**, *108*, 103629. [CrossRef] [PubMed]
22. Cumbo, E.; Scardina, G.A. Management and use of filter masks in the "none-medical" population during the COVID-19 period. *Saf. Sci.* **2021**, *133*, 104997. [CrossRef] [PubMed]
23. Jakubowski, A.; Egger, D.; Nekesa, C.; Lowe, L.; Walker, M.; Miguel, E. Self-reported vs directly observed face mask use in Kenya. *JAMA Netw. Open* **2021**, *4*, e2118830. [CrossRef] [PubMed]
24. Dryhurst, S.; Schneider, C.R.; Kerr, J.; Freeman, A.L.; Recchia, G.; Van Der Bles, A.M.; Spiegelhalter, D.; Van Der Linden, S. Risk perceptions of COVID-19 around the world. *J. Risk Res.* **2020**, *23*, 994–1006. [CrossRef]
25. Chughtai, A.A.; Seale, H.; MacIntyre, C.R. Use of cloth masks in the practice of infection control evidence and policy gaps. *Int. J. Infect. Control* **2013**, *9*, 1–12. [CrossRef]
26. MacIntyre, C.R.; Seale, H.; Dung, T.C.; Hien, N.T.; Nga, P.T.; Chughtai, A.A.; Rahman, B.; Dwyer, D.E.; Wang, Q. A cluster randomised trial of cloth masks compared with medical masks in healthcare workers. *BMJ Open* **2015**, *5*, e006577. [CrossRef]
27. Grinshpun, S.A.; Haruta, H.; Eninger, R.M.; Reponen, T.; McKay, R.T.; Lee, S.A. Performance of an N95 Filtering Facepiece Particulate Respirator and a Surgical Mask During Human Breathing: Two Pathways for Particle Penetration. *J. Occup. Environ. Hyg.* **2009**, *6*, 593–603. [CrossRef]
28. Guellich, A.; Tella, E.; Ariane, M.; Grodner, C.; Nguyen-Chi, H.N.; Mahé, E. The face mask-touching behavior during the COVID-19 pandemic: Observational study of public transportation users in the greater Paris region: The French-mask-touch study. *J. Transp. Health* **2021**, *21*, 101078. [CrossRef]
29. Kellerer, J.D.; Rohringer, M.; Deufert, D. Behavior in the use of face masks in the context of COVID-19. *Public Health Nurs.* **2021**, *38*, 862–868. [CrossRef]
30. Howard, J.; Huang, A.; Li, Z.; Tufekci, Z.; Zdimal, V.; van der Westhuizen, H.M.; von Delft, A.; Price, A.; Fridman, L.; Tang, L.H.; et al. An evidence review of face masks against COVID-19. *Proc. Natl. Acad. Sci. USA* **2021**, *118*, e2014564118. [CrossRef]
31. Au, T.K.; Chan, C.K.; Chan, T.K.; Cheung, M.W.; Ho, J.Y.; Ip, G.W. Folkbiology meets microbiology: A study of conceptual and behavioral change. *Cogn. Psychol.* **2008**, *57*, 1–9. [CrossRef] [PubMed]

International Journal of
Environmental Research and Public Health

MDPI

Article

COVID-19 Vaccinating Russian Medical Students—Challenges and Solutions: A Cross-Sectional Study

Olesya V. Kytko [1], Yuriy L. Vasil'ev [1], Sergey S. Dydykin [1], Ekaterina Yu Diachkova [1,*], Maria V. Sankova [1], Tatiana M. Litvinova [1], Beatrice A. Volel [1], Kirill A. Zhandarov [1], Andrey A. Grishin [1], Vladislav V. Tatarkin [2], Dmitriy E. Suetenkov [3], Alexander I. Nikolaev [4], Michael Yu Pastbin [5], Innokenty D. Ushnitsky [6], Svetlana N. Gromova [7], Gulshat T. Saleeva [8], Liaisan Saleeva [8], Nail Saleev [8], Eduard Shakirov [8] and Rinat A. Saleev [8]

1 Sklifosovskyi Institute of Clinical Medicine, I.M. Sechenov First Moscow State Medical University, St. Trubetskaya, 8, bld. 2, 119991 Moscow, Russia
2 Department of Operative and Clinical Surgery with Topographic Anatomy Named after S.A. Simbirtsev, Mechnikov North-West State Medical University, Kirochnaya St., 41, 191015 Saint-Petersburg, Russia
3 Department of Pediatric Dentistry and Orthodontics, V.I. Razumovsky Saratov State Medical University, B. Kazachya St., 112, 410012 Saratov, Russia
4 Department of Therapeutic Dentistry, Smolensk State Medical University, Krupskoy St., 28, 214019 Smolensk, Russia
5 Department of Children Dentistry, Northern State Medical University, Troitsky Avenue, 51, 163000 Arkhangelsk, Russia
6 Department of Therapeutic, Surgical and Prosthetic Dentistry, M.K. Ammosov North-Eastern Federal University, Belinsky St., 58, 677000 Yakutsk, Russia
7 Department of Dentistry, Kirov State Medical University, K. Marx St., d.112, 610998 Kirov, Russia
8 Department of Prosthetic Dentistry, Kazan State Medical University, Butlerova St., 49, 420012 Kazan, Russia
* Correspondence: secu2003@mail.ru

Citation: Kytko, O.V.; Vasil'ev, Y.L.; Dydykin, S.S.; Diachkova, E.Y.; Sankova, M.V.; Litvinova, T.M.; Volel, B.A.; Zhandarov, K.A.; Grishin, A.A.; Tatarkin, V.V.; et al. COVID-19 Vaccinating Russian Medical Students—Challenges and Solutions: A Cross-Sectional Study. *Int. J. Environ. Res. Public Health* **2022**, *19*, 11556. https://doi.org/10.3390/ijerph191811556

Academic Editor: Giuseppe Alessandro Scardina

Received: 23 July 2022
Accepted: 9 September 2022
Published: 14 September 2022

Abstract: *Background*: The role of preventive measures increases significantly in the absence of effective specific COVID-19 treatment. Mass population immunization and the achievement of collective immunity are of particular importance. The future development of public attitudes towards SARS-CoV-2 immunization depends significantly on medical students, as future physicians. Therefore, it seemed relevant to determine the percentage of COVID-19-vaccinated medical students and to identify the factors significantly affecting this indicator. *Methods*: A total of 2890 medical students from years one to six, studying at nine leading Russian medical universities, participated in an anonymous sociological survey. The study was performed in accordance with the STROBE guidelines. *Results:* It was found that the percentage of vaccinated Russian medical students at the beginning of the academic year 2021 was 58.8 ± 7.69%, which did not significantly differ from the vaccination coverage of the general population in the corresponding regions (54.19 ± 4.83%). Student vaccination rate was largely determined by the region-specific epidemiological situation. The level of student vaccination coverage did not depend on the gender or student residence (in a family or in a university dormitory). The group of senior students had a higher number of COVID-19 vaccine completers than the group of junior students. The lack of reliable information about COVID-19 vaccines had a pronounced negative impact on the SARS-CoV-2 immunization process. Significant information sources influencing student attitudes toward vaccination included medical professionals, medical universities, academic conferences, and manuscripts, which at that time provided the least information. *Conclusion:* The obtained results make it possible to develop recommendations to promote SARS-CoV-2 immunoprophylaxis among students and the general population and to increase collective immunity.

Keywords: COVID-19 pandemic; COVID-19 vaccination coverage; COVID-19 vaccination problems; epidemiological indicators; medical students; SARS-CoV-2 immunoprophylaxis

1. Introduction

The long-term pandemic of the new coronavirus infection caused by the single-stranded RNA-containing virus SARS-CoV-2 has become a serious challenge not only for the healthcare systems but also for the economies of all countries [1]. Unprecedented measures are being taken to organize medical care for SARS-CoV-2-infected people and to rehabilitate patients with severe post-COVID complications [2]. In the absence of effective specific COVID-19 treatment, the role of prophylaxis increases significantly. Along with nonspecific prevention methods and compliance with sanitary–epidemiological requirements, mass population immunization and the achievement of collective immunity are of particular importance [3,4].

Over the years of the pandemic, a significant amount of scientific information has been accumulated on the SARS-CoV-2 pathogenesis, the virus biology, and its interaction with the human immune system, making it possible to create effective COVID-19 vaccines [5–7]. In Russia, the first COVID-19 vaccine was officially recognized in August 2020. It was the two-component "Gam-COVID-Vac" ("Sputnik V"), based on the safe rAD26-S и rAD5-S adenovirus carriers and developed by the N.F. Gamaleya Federal Research Center for Epidemiology & Microbiology. The main advantage of such viral vector vaccines is their natural mechanism of transporting SARS-CoV-2 genetic fragments into human cells, allowing for sufficient long-term antigen expression, effectively activating innate and adaptive immunity [8–10]. Then, in October 2020, the genetically engineered protein vaccine "EpiVacCorona", made from three different artificial peptides copying SARS-CoV-2 fragments, was registered by the by State Research Center of Virology and Biotechnology "Vector". Persons over 18 years of age without contraindications are allowed to be vaccinated with the "Sputnik V" and "EpiVacCorona" vaccines [11,12]. The most traditional technological platform for creating vaccines was used by the Chumakov Federal Scientific Center for Research and Development of Immune and Biological Products of the Russian Academy of Sciences, which developed an inactivated whole-virion vaccine, "CoviVak", that became available in February 2021 for persons from 18 to 60 [13–16]. All these vaccines are administered twice intramuscularly at 2–3 weeks' interval [8,10,12,17–19]. In May 2021 the first component of the "Sputnik V" vaccine was registered as "Sputnik Light", which was intended for revaccination or vaccination of young people (18–30 years old), whose immunity is well formed, and one injection is enough. Later, "EpiVacCorona" was optimized into "EpiVacCorona H", in which two of the three peptides were combined into one [9,10,19–25]. In Moscow, COVID-19 vaccination began on 5 December 2020; in other Russian regions, this was on 10 December, according to the unified COVID-19 immunization program. Military, teachers, health care workers, and social workers were the first in the vaccination campaign. SARS-CoV-2 immunization became available to everyone in Russia in January 2021. Persons who have completed the full COVID-19 vaccination course receive a special certificate that is required in order to be able to visit public places and educational institutions [9–11,13–15].

A special risk group in the pandemic situation is medical students who have a high infection risk due to their frequent visits to different patients and emergency practice in coronavirus hospitals [26–28]. Medical students, as future physicians, are essential in forming public attitudes towards SARS-CoV-2 immunization since there is currently a worldwide problem of insufficient vaccination coverage due to mistrust and deliberate avoidance of this highly effective measure [29]. In this regard, it was particularly important to study the real COVID-19 vaccination rates among medical students during the SARS-CoV-2 pandemic. The goal of this study was to determine the percentage of COVID-19-vaccinated medical students and to identify the factors that significantly affect this indicator in order to be able to develop recommendations that will help to increase vaccination rates among the population and achieve the target of collective immunity.

2. Materials and Methods

2.1. Study Design and Participants

A total of 2890 1st- to 6th-year medical students from nine leading Russian universities located in the regions with different epidemiological SARS-CoV-2 situation were included in a cross-sectional online anonymous survey conducted in the period of late September—early October 2021 (Figure 1). By this time, students had had the opportunity to be vaccinated against COVID-19 for more than six months from the start of vaccination.

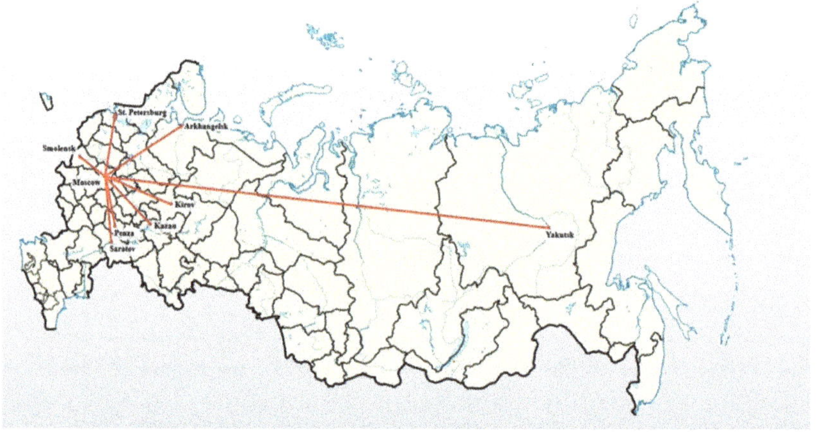

Figure 1. Regions of online medical student survey in Russia.

The study was carried out on the Google Forms platform (Alphabet, Mountain View, California, USA) in accordance with STROBE guidelines. The reference to the questionnaire was distributed among students through social networks and Internet information channels. Using G*Power software statistical package (ChristianAlbrechts-Universität, Olshausenstr, Germany) [30] and based on a moderate effect size 0.3, power 85%, and alpha < 0.05, the minimum sample size needed for this study was calculated to equal 1706 student that was approximately 7.52% of the total number of students (22,694 students) enrolled in the nine institutes. The formula used and the calculations for the minimum sample size are shown below (Figure 2).

$$N = \frac{p_0 q_0 \left\{ z_{1-\alpha/2} + z_{1-\beta} \sqrt{\frac{p_1 q_1}{p_0 q_0}} \right\}^2}{(p_1 - p_0)^2}$$

$$q_0 = 1 - p_0$$

$$q_1 = 1 - p_1$$

(**a**)

$$N = \frac{0.06 * 0.94 \left\{ 1.96 + 1.04 \sqrt{\frac{0.078 * 0.922}{0.06 * 0.94}} \right\}^2}{(0.078 - 0.06)^2}$$

$$N = 1706$$

(**b**)

Figure 2. Sample size count: (**a**) 'classic' formula for counting; (**b**) formula and counting process for present study.

Respondent sample representativeness in each of the nine universities is presented in Table 1.

Table 1. Number and percentage of surveyed medical students.

Russian Higher Education Institution	Number and Percentage of Respondents	Total Number of Students
I.M. Sechenov First Moscow State Medical University (Sechenov University)	575 (13.2%)	4356
Mechnikov North-West State Medical University	302 (10.8%)	2797
Saratov State Medical University named after V.I. Razumovsky (Razumovsky University)	283 (12.9%)	2194
Smolensk State Medical University	215 (12.6%)	1707
Northern State Medical University	290 (11.7%)	2479
Federal State Autonomous Educational Institution of Higher Education "M. K. Ammosov North-Eastern Federal University"	212 (11.5%)	1845
Kirov State Medical University	344 (13.6%)	2529
Kazan State Medical University	469 (15.1%)	3106
Penza State Medical University	200 (11.9%)	1681
Total	2890 (12.7%)	22,694

2.2. *Epidemiological Situation Characteristics in Studied Russian Regions*

The up-to-date data provided by Russian Federal Service on Customers' Rights Protection and Human Well-Being Surveillance (Russian Federal Service on Customers' Rights Protection and Human Well-Being Surveillance—the up-to-date data are available at: https://xn--80aesfpebagmfblc0a.xn--p1ai/information/, accessed on 15 November 2021) were used to identify the correlation between student behavioral attitudes toward SARS-CoV-2 immunization in relation to morbidity, mortality, lethality, and vaccination population coverage of the corresponding Russian region.

Moscow and Saint Petersburg led steadily with respect to numbers of patients and number of deaths per 1000 people among the Russian regions studied ($p < 0.05$). Minimum incidence and mortality were observed in the Tatarstan Republic ($p < 0.05$), where Kazan State Medical University is located (Figures 3 and 4).

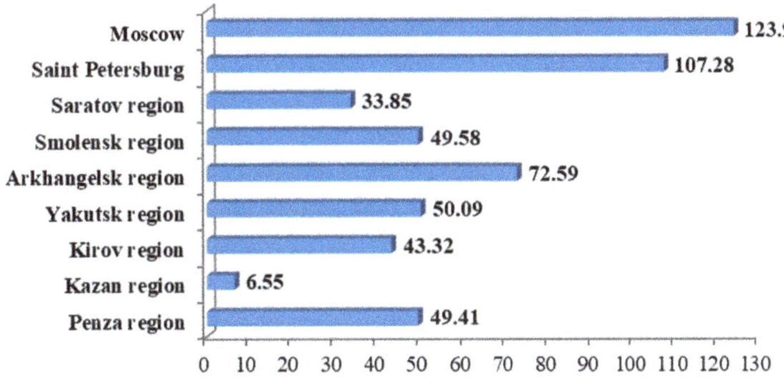

Figure 3. Total SARS-CoV-2 incidence per 1000 people at the time of the study.

The highest lethality rates, defined as the ratio of deaths occurring because of SARS-CoV-2 to the total number of people affected by the disease during the pandemic period, were recorded in Saint Petersburg, Penza, and Smolensk regions ($p < 0.05$). The minimum value of this indicator was observed in the Kirov region ($p < 0.05$) (Figure 5).

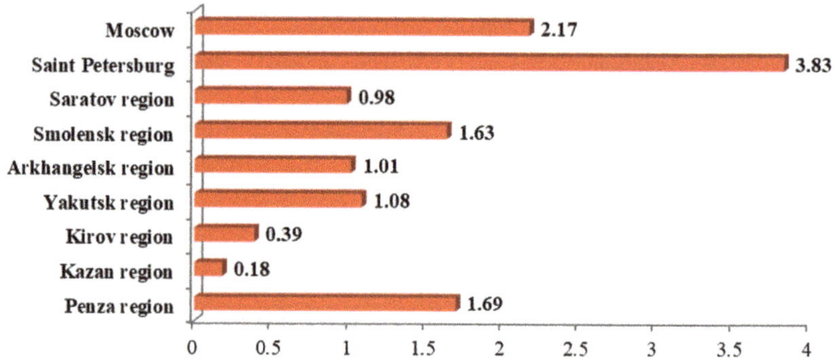

Figure 4. Total mortality because of SARS-CoV-2 per 1000 people at the time of the study.

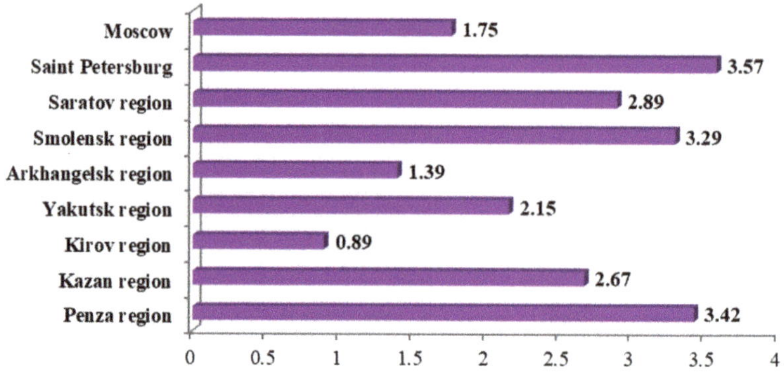

Figure 5. Lethality because of SARS-CoV-2 at the time of the study.

COVID-19 vaccination coverage of the population of each region at the time of the study is shown in Figure 6. It should be emphasized that the proportion of vaccinated people in Moscow, Smolensk and Arkhangelsk regions was significantly lower than in the Tatarstan Republic, Kirov and Penza regions. On average, the percentage of citizens that had been vaccinated in the studied regions was 54.1%, while in the whole of Russia this figure was 52.3%.

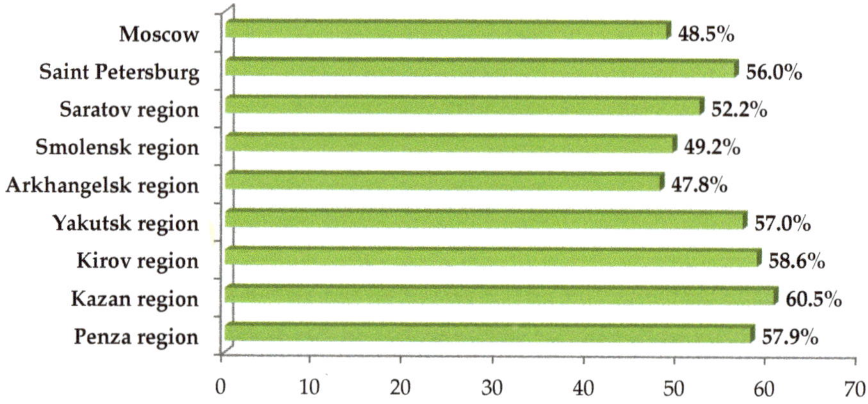

Figure 6. Vaccination coverage of the populations of the studied regions at the time of the study.

2.3. Questionnaire Development and Content

The original questionnaire was designed using prior scientific studies on vaccine and behavioral attitudes toward immunization, with new factors added [26–28,31–35]. Personal information such as institutional affiliation, academic year, student residence, age, and sex were requested to be filled in first (Supplementary Materials). The main part of the questionnaire consisted of four sections, the first of which contained questions about COVID-19 assessment, previous COVID-19 experience in relatives and themselves, attitudes towards non-specific SARS-CoV-2 preventive measures, and the evaluation of their effectiveness. In the second section, student beliefs about COVID-19 vaccination were studied. To identify their determination of the effectiveness of vaccination and non-specific SARS-CoV-2 preventive measures, students used a visual analog scale, in which 10 points corresponded to the effectiveness maximum, and 0 points to its complete absence. The third section focuses on participant COVID-19 vaccine preference and vaccine information sources. Finally, we investigated COVID-19 vaccination coverage among medical students, side effects after COVID-19 vaccination, and predominant reasons for not vaccinating. In the final questions, respondents were able to choose several options. To ensure questionnaire content validity, a pilot study was carried out on 36 students who were not included in the final study. All questions were checked for clarity and ease of understanding by three independent experienced experts.

2.4. Ethical Considerations

The work fully complied with the requirements of the local ethical committee of Sechenov University (Protocol No. 04-19 dated 6 March 2019) and the norms of the Declaration of Helsinki. All students were recruited on a volunteer basis and gave informed consent before the study. Respondents understood the survey purpose and were told how to fill in the questionnaire. No reward was offered to participants.

2.5. Statistical Analysis

Statistical data analysis was performed using SPSS 20.0 (SPSS Inc., Chicago, IL, USA) and MedCalc 11.5.00 (MedCalc Software, Oostende, Belgium). The minimal subject number needed for this study was calculated by means of power analysis. Descriptive statistics had a place for data from scales where the mean, median, standard deviation, and percentiles were calculated. Intergroup qualitative indicators were compared using Pearson's χ-squared test or Fisher's exact test. The normality of distributions was checked with Kolmogorov–Smirnov test. Quantitative differences were determined using the independent t-test for normal distribution or the non-parametric Mann–Whitney U-test when variables were non-normally distributed. For multiple-comparison, non-parametric Kruskal–Wallis test and parametric ANOVA were used. Pearson's coefficient and Spearman's rank test were calculated for correlation analysis. Statistics were considered significant at $p < 0.05$. The results were counted twice by 2 independent researchers. The inter- and intragroup correlation agreement rates were greater than 95%; for this reason, all results were considered as the mean between 2 attempts by 2 researchers.

3. Results

3.1. Participant Characteristics

The mean respondent age was 20.99 ± 2.28 years (range of 16 to 37 years) (Table 2). The survey sample included students from the 1st to 6th year; therefore, two subgroups of junior (1–3 year—1467 (50.8%)) and senior (4–6 year—1423 (49.2%)) students were formed to determine the dependence of commitment to COVID-19 vaccination on the professional training level. There were 800 males (27.7%) and 2090 females (72.3%), which was used to examine the proportion vaccinated according to sex.

Table 2. Mean age of surveyed medical students and their number according to sex and grade.

Russian Higher Education Institution	Mean Age	1–3 Year	4–6 Year	Males	Females
I.M. Sechenov First Moscow State Medical University (Sechenov University)	19.53 ± 3.01	299	276	133	442
Mechnikov North-West State Medical University	19.96 ± 2.32	162	140	75	227
Saratov State Medical University named after V.I. Razumovsky (Razumovsky University)	19.65 ± 2.64	157	126	80	203
Smolensk State Medical University	20.81 ± 2.13	84	131	67	148
Northern State Medical University	21.49 ± 1.96	127	163	62	228
Federal State Autonomous Educational Institution of Higher Education "M. K. Ammosov North-Eastern Federal University"	22.88 ± 3.67	108	104	84	128
Kirov State Medical University	22.05 ± 2.56	170	174	88	256
Kazan State Medical University	20.47 ± 2.46	277	192	141	328
Penza State Medical University	22.10 ± 1.79	83	117	70	130
Total	20.99 ± 2.28	1467 (50.8%)	1423 (49.2%)	800 (27.7%)	2090 (72.3%)

3.2. *Participant COVID-19 Experience and Non-Specific SARS-CoV-2 Prophylaxis Evaluation*

Most students consider COVID-19 a dangerous disease (89.4%) and express profound concern about the current unfavorable sanitary–epidemiological situation (89.9%) associated with the rapid spread of new coronavirus variants. Three-quarters of the respondents have already encountered this disease in their relatives (75.9%), and every third had experienced the death of a loved one (36.98 ± 5.79%). Almost half of the young surveyed people (48.6%) had experienced RT-PCR test-confirmed COVID-19 themselves, with one in two (46.6%) being diagnosed with moderate and severe form of this disease (according to computed tomography criteria). Most students (85.4%) are responsible with respect to following non-specific SARS-CoV-2 preventive measures, which primarily include wearing masks in public places, treating hands with antiseptic, and social distancing. Respondents rated the effectiveness of these anti-COVID measures at 4.73 ± 0.51 points (the median was 5.0 (IQR, 3.0–7.0).

3.3. *Participant Beliefs about COVID-19 Vaccination*

Most future specialists (65.0%) consider vaccination to be the most effective method for infectious disease prevention; every second respondent (57.3%) sees the immunization expediency even directly during a pandemic. However, only a little more than a third of all students (39.0%) expressed a definite positive attitude towards COVID-19 vaccination, and the same number of respondents (42.7%) have not yet fully decided on this issue, so only half of all respondents (52.5%) recommend their relatives, friends, and acquaintances to vaccinate against coronavirus infection.

The effectiveness of SARS-CoV-2 specific prophylaxis was estimated by medical students at 4.87 ± 0.50 points (the median was 5.0 (IQR, 3.0–7.0), which did not differ significantly from the effectiveness of non-specific SARS-CoV-2 preventive measures (4.73 ± 0.51, respectively; $p > 0.05$). Many future doctors (66.5%) believe that COVID-19 vaccine prophylaxis acts as a necessary guarantee of protection against moderate and severe disease forms, fatal outcomes, and post-infectious complications. Only a tenth of the respondents (10.9%) suppose that active immunization can prevent disease incidence.

Just over half of the students (59.2%) indicate that the COVID-19 vaccination need is primarily for at-risk individuals and adults. A quarter of respondents note that both adults and children should be vaccinated. One in six students (14.7%) is convinced that SARS-CoV-2 immunization is not indicated for anyone at all (Figure 7). Almost all students (86.5%) emphasize that vaccination should be voluntary only.

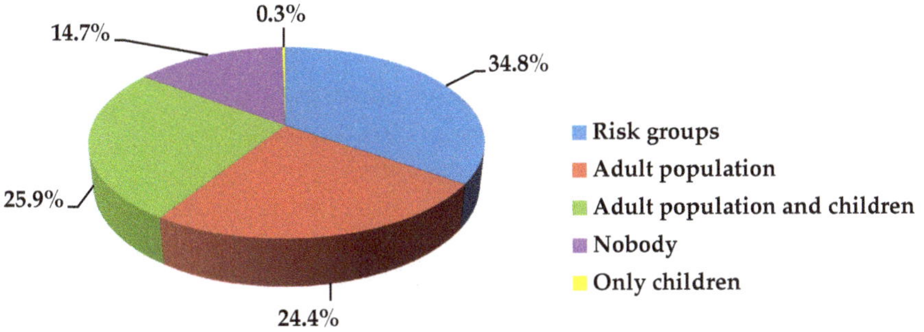

Figure 7. Population groups to be vaccinated against COVID-19.

3.4. Participant COVID-19 Vaccine Preference and Vaccine Information Sources

The highest percentage of (41.9%) medical students express the opinion that all COVID-19 vaccines are effective regardless of the origin country, 18.3% respondents are convinced of the good quality of only Russian vaccines, 24.3% respondents trust only imported vaccines. Every sixth medical student (15.5%) believes that all immunobiological agents are ineffective.

Every third medical school student (31.9%) reported a clear lack of reliable information about anti-COVID vaccines, their composition, action mechanisms and contraindications. Sources of COVID-19 preventive vaccines, used by medical students for subsequent informed consent or refusal to participate in a vaccination campaign against COVID-19, were identified (Figure 8).

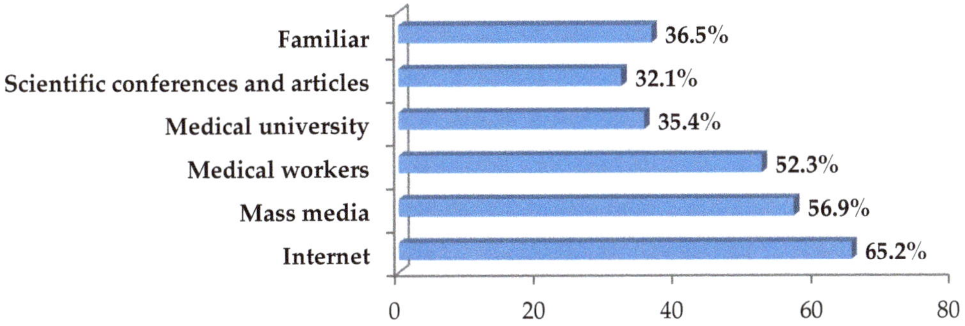

Figure 8. Key information sources of COVID-19 vaccines in medical students.

Thus, medical students received most information about active SARS-CoV-2 immunization drugs from the Internet and the mass media. Half of the respondents, in order to make their choice (52.3%), relied on information obtained from medical professionals. The least importance in obtaining knowledge about vaccines was found for medical universities, scientific conferences and manuscripts, the role of which is reported only by a third of students, which is comparable to the number of students whose source of information is familiar. Half of future doctors (47.7%) are not satisfied with the quality of information they received at all.

3.5. COVID-19 Vaccination among Medical Students and Reasons for Not Vaccinating

The COVID-19 vaccination coverage among Russian medical students was 58.8%, which did not significantly differ from the percentage of citizens who were vaccinated in the studied regions, which was 54.2% ($p < 0.05$). The distribution of the vaccinated by the region in Russia is shown in Figure 9. It should be noted that the percentage of preventive

COVID-19 vaccination among the students of Saratov, Kirov and Northern State Medical University is significantly lower than that at other universities ($p < 0.05$).

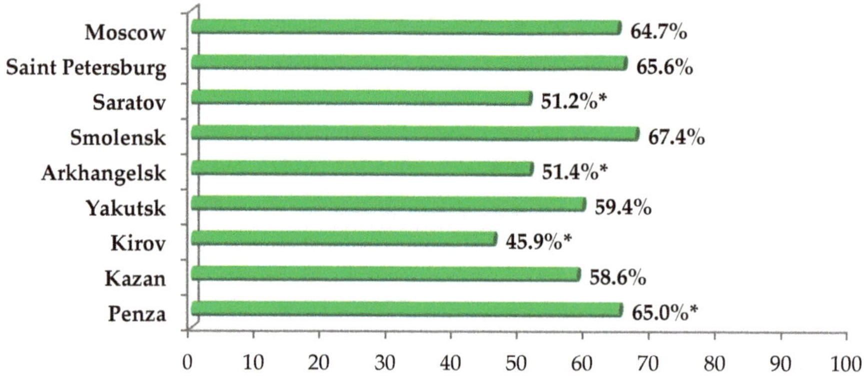

Figure 9. The distribution of vaccinated medical students by Russian region. Note: *—the differences are significant, $p < 0.05$.

The percentage of COVID-19-vaccinated students was not dependent on gender (57.9% and 61.3%, respectively; $p > 0.05$), and was significantly higher in the group of senior students compared to junior students (68.7% and 49.2%, respectively; $p < 0.05$). It was found that in a significantly larger percentage of cases, students were motivated to receive the COVID-19 vaccination certificate than to prevent the disease and its severe course (59.2% and 45.4%, respectively; $p < 0.05$).

The most popular vaccines chosen by medical students for the SARS-CoV-2 prevention were the combined two-component vaccine "Gam-COVID-Vac" ("Sputnik V") and the single-component vaccine Sputnik-Light, based on viral vectors and developed by the N.F. Gamaleya Federal Research Center for Epidemiology & Microbiology (Figure 10). In second place was the medication "CoviVak", an inactivated whole-virion vaccine, registered by the Chumakov Federal Scientific Center for Research and Development of Immune and Biological Products of Russian Academy of Sciences. The subunit (protein) vaccines "EpiVacCorona" and "EpiVacCorona H", developed by the by State Research Center of Virology and Biotechnology "Vector", were the least in demand.

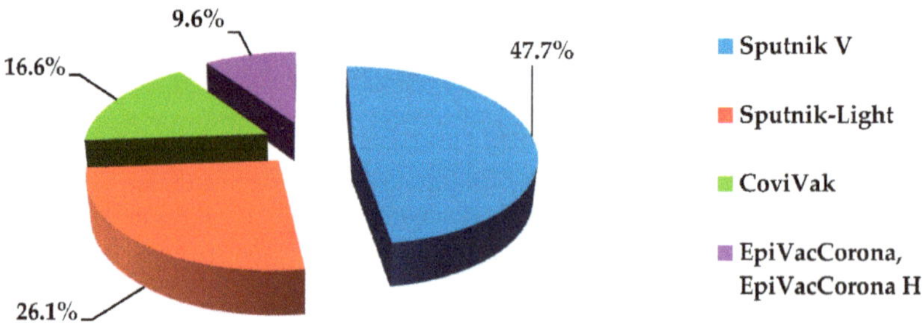

Figure 10. COVID-19 vaccines selected by medical students.

The most common side effects after COVID-19 vaccination were weakness (71.4%), injection site soreness (66.2%), fever (64.5%), headache (54.1%) and muscle aches (52.2%), which, as a rule, disappeared on their own within 2–3 days. In 14.8% of respondents, side effects were completely absent.

The predominant reasons for not vaccinating were lack of awareness about COVID-19 vaccines and doubts about their efficacy and safety (15.3%), fear of side effects and post-vaccination complications (23.5%), presence of post-COVID immunity (15.3%) and medical withdrawal from vaccination due to existing contraindications (12.0%).

3.6. Identifying Factors Affecting COVID-19 Vaccination Coverage among Medical Students

Multicomponent correlation analysis made it possible to identify the factors affecting the COVID-19 vaccination coverage among Russian medical students. Thus, it was shown that the student attitude towards COVID-19 vaccination was almost independent of their opinion about the danger of this coronavirus infection (r = −0.009) and their concern about the current sanitary–epidemiological situation (r = −0.235). It was found that students were motivated to carry out specific prophylaxis not so much by an increase in the overall incidence in the region (r = 0.388) as by the incidence among students themselves (r = 0.573) and their relatives (r = 0.626). Increased mortality rates because of SARS-CoV-2 (r = 0.655) and, especially, the percentage of deaths among close people (r = 0.778) had a great effect. It should be noted that there is a strong positive correlation between the percentage of vaccinated medical students and the lethality rate because of SARS-CoV-2 in this region (r = 0.701). There was no relationship between the SARS-CoV-2 immunization coverage of the region population and the proportion of SARS-CoV-2 vaccinated medical students (r = −0.119).

A pronounced negative impact on the SARS-CoV-2 immunization process was provided by the lack of information about COVID-19 vaccines (r = −0.638) and the unreliability of these data (r = −0.693), which determine the doubt about the vaccination effectiveness and safety (r = 0.674), and the fear of side effects and post-vaccination complications (r = 0.686). It was found that the percentage of students who decided to be vaccinated against SARS-CoV-2 was positively correlated with the percentage of students whose main information sources were medical professionals (r = 0.484), medical university (r = 0.584), and scientific conferences and manuscripts (r = 0.317). Information from the Internet (r = 0.164) and from familiar (r = −0.096) had no significant effect on student SARS-CoV-2 immunization attitudes. Students who received information mainly from the mass media vaccinated in a significantly lower percentage (r = −0.623). It should be emphasized that the percentage of young people who were negative about SARS-CoV-2 immunization (r = −0.450) and not fully decided on this issue (r = −0.722) was negatively correlated with the percentage of COVID-19-vaccinated students.

It was found that the student COVID-19 vaccination coverage did not depend on their student residence, i.e., whether they lived in a family (r = 0.055) or in a university dormitory (r = −0.043). A negative correlation was noted between the percentage of COVID-19-vaccinated students and the proportion of students who exclusively prefer foreign vaccines (r = −0.322). The percentage of future specialists who recommended COVID-19 vaccination to everyone around them and who, accordingly, largely affect the formation of collective population immunity, was significantly correlated with the percentage of students who were positive about SARS-CoV-2 immunization and had been vaccinated themselves (r = 0.903).

Study design and research results are summed up in flow chart diagram (Figure S1—Supplementary Materials).

4. Discussion

According to recent studies, the understanding of the importance of the COVID-19 vaccine among medical students all over the world is very high, since COVID is a potentially severe acute respiratory infection [28,36–39]. However, the presence of words such as 'hesitancy', 'barriers', and 'refusal' in the literature regarding COVID-19 vaccination demonstrates the clear problems of COVID-19 vaccine approval among the young medical community. It was shown that almost all Russian medical students believed that COVID-19 was a serious disease (89.3%) and expressed profound concern about the current epidemiological situation (89.9%), sounding similar to the common understanding of the situation among medical students from around the world; vaccination importance was recognized by most of the respondents in the known studies, reaching 73.2–99.4% [36–39].

Hesitancy in accepting COVID-19 vaccination has a place among medical students in different countries and in some studies its prevalence even reaches 23.0–46.0% [27,28,40]. In Russia, most future specialists (65.0%) consider active population immunization to be the most effective method of preventing infectious diseases and post-infectious complications, but only a third of them (39.0%) have a positive attitude towards COVID-19 vaccination, and 42.7% of respondents are still undecided on this issue, and show low intention to recommend COVID-19 vaccination to others (demonstration of 'hesitancy'). This criterion does not exactly exceed the percentage reported in other studies, but it is very close to the highest negative level. The need to obtain COVID-19 vaccination certificates motivated students to get vaccinated more than the desire to prevent COVID-19 and its complications.

Therefore, the real COVID-19 vaccination rate among Russian medical students in autumn 2021 was shown to be 58.8 $\pm$ 7.69%, which did not differ from the COVID-19 vaccination coverage among the general population at that time, and was significantly lower than the target value for collective immunity, which, according to actual data of the Russian Federal Service on Customers' Rights Protection and Human Well-Being Surveillance was 80%. The number of COVID-19-vaccinated medical students worldwide was also not sufficient and according to systematic analysis of 40 original articles published between January 2020 and December 2021 averaged 61.9% [41].

It was found that the main reason for COVID-19 vaccination hesitancy among medical students and the low vaccination rate in Russia is the lack of reliable information on COVID-19 vaccines, their composition, action mechanisms and contraindications, which determine the doubt about the effectiveness and safety of COVID-19 vaccination, and the fear of side effects and post-vaccination complications, which has also been emphasized by other scientists [28,33,34]. It has been proved that the percentage of students who decided to be vaccinated against SARS-CoV-2 was positively correlated with the percentage of students whose main sources of information were medical professionals, medical universities, scientific conferences, and manuscripts, which at that point provided the least information about active SARS-CoV-2 immunization to medical students. Students who received data mainly from the media were vaccinated in a significantly lower percentage because of anti-vaccination propaganda conducted there. Similar assumptions were made in other studies [28,36]. Lack of information about COVID-19 vaccines can be a source of stress for young medical specialists [42].

For the first time, it was found that the student COVID-19 vaccination rate was largely determined by the actual epidemiological situation of the region, and primarily by indicators such as mortality ($r = 0.655$) and lethality ($r = 0.701$), which may be related to medical students' awareness of COVID-19 treatment options and care quality in corresponding regions. It was proved that student COVID-19 vaccination coverage rates were independent of gender and student residence. For the first time, our study demonstrated that the group of senior students had a higher number of COVID-19 vaccine completers than the group of junior students, which may be due to their greater involvement in coronavirus hospitals and more frequent contact with health care workers. Other authors also established that willingness to be vaccinated against COVID-19 among medical students generally increased with age and education [27].

It has been shown that the percentage of students willing to recommend COVID-19 vaccination to the people around them and thereby contribute to increasing the collective immunity level is significantly dependent on the percentage of students who have been COVID-19 vaccinated. Many scientists consider that medical students are among the front-line medical professionals who meet patients. In addition, it is very important to achieve high rates of COVID-19 vaccination coverage in this group of health care providers, as they will recommend COVID-19 vaccination and counsel vaccine-hesitant people [27]. Public attitudes toward COVID-19 vaccine prophylaxis are formed in communication with medical students and directly depend on their competence in this matter. The ability to competently convey to the patient the essence of SARS-CoV-2 immunologic prophylaxis, to justify its necessity, to explain the existing questions in an accessible language, to inform about possible adverse reactions are the most important student skills, which they should receive, first, at a medical university.

One of our study limitations was the lack of result separation by faculty, as there is a perception that medical student knowledge varies between different specializations. We consider all respondents to have a high level of education corresponding to their course. In addition, the relatively small number of males compared to females may likely be a limiting factor on the study results. In future studies we will choose proportional numbers of students from all medical universities. Another limitation is that the survey was conducted under the condition that only Russian vaccines were included. For this reason, this study and its results must be understood as the initial stage of multi-central research for COVID-19 vaccination in order to understand its problems.

5. Conclusions

The real COVID-19 vaccination rate among Russian medical students in autumn 2021 was 58.8 ± 7.69%, which did not differ from the COVID-19 vaccination coverage of the general population at that time, and was significantly lower than the target value for collective immunity. The main reason for low COVID-19 vaccination among medical students' rate is the lack of reliable information about COVID-19 vaccines. Significant information sources influencing students' attitudes toward vaccination include medical professionals, medical universities, academic conferences, and manuscripts. The group of senior students had a higher number of COVID-19 vaccine completers than the group of junior students.

The obtained results support the following recommendations:

(1) The primary task is to eliminate the information deficiency about COVID-19 vaccines among medical students using educational resources and, above all, the medical university, considering its significance in the forming adherence to SARS-CoV-2 immunologic prophylaxis. (2) SARS-CoV-2 immunologic prophylaxis education should be organized to all students, focusing on junior students. (3) Registration of foreign COVID-19 vaccines in Russia and development of official recommendations for their use will increase the percentage of vaccinated students and population. (4) A conscious decision by medical students to be vaccinated against SARS-CoV-2 will contribute to their competent explanation of immunologic prophylaxis essence to the population and increase collective immunity.

Supplementary Materials: The following supporting information can be downloaded at: https://www.mdpi.com/article/10.3390/ijerph191811556/s1, Figure S1. Flow research chart.

Author Contributions: Conceptualization, O.V.K., M.V.S., B.A.V. and S.S.D.; methodology, Y.L.V., M.V.S., B.A.V., K.A.Z. and L.S.; resources, A.A.G., O.V.K., V.V.T., D.E.S., A.I.N., M.Y.P., I.D.U., S.N.G., R.A.S. and G.T.S.; data analysis, M.V.S., E.Y.D. and E.S.; writing—original draft preparation, M.V.S. and O.V.K.; writing—review and editing, M.V.S., E.Y.D. and K.A.Z.; project administration O.V.K., Y.L.V. and T.M.L.; Formal analysis, N.S. All authors have read and agreed to the published version of the manuscript.

Funding: The research is supported by Scientific program 'Prioritet-2030'.

Institutional Review Board Statement: Current research study was approved by the Ethics Committee of First Moscow State Medical University named after I.M. Sechenov (Sechenov University) under protocol N° 04-19 dated 6 March 2019.

Informed Consent Statement: Informed consent was obtained from all subjects involved in the study.

Data Availability Statement: The data are not publicly available due to Local Ethical Committee requirements.

Acknowledgments: We thanks all participants and Universities for help in the study conduction.

Conflicts of Interest: The authors declare no conflict of interest in the writing and preparation of this article.

References

1. Trovato, M.; Sartorius, R.; D'Apice, L.; Manco, R.; De Berardinis, P. Viral Emerging Diseases: Challenges in Developing Vaccination Strategies. *Front. Immunol.* **2020**, *11*, 2130. [CrossRef] [PubMed]
2. Wosik, J.; Fudim, M.; Cameron, B.; Gellad, Z.F.; Cho, A.; Phinney, D.; Curtis, S.; Roman, M.; Poon, E.G.; Ferranti, J.; et al. Telehealth transformation: COVID-19 and the rise of virtual care. *J. Am. Med. Inform. Assoc.* **2020**, *27*, 957–962. [CrossRef] [PubMed]
3. Velikova, T.; Georgiev, T. SARS-CoV-2 vaccines and autoimmune diseases amidst the COVID-19 crisis. *Rheumatol. Int.* **2021**, *41*, 509–518. [CrossRef] [PubMed]
4. Štefan, M.; Dlouhý, P.; Bezdíčková, L. Vaccination against COVID-19. *Klin. Mikrobiol. Infekc Lek.* **2021**, *27*, 49–60. [PubMed]
5. Castells, M.C.; Phillips, E.J. Maintaining Safety with SARS-CoV-2 Vaccines. *N. Engl. J. Med.* **2021**, *384*, 643–649. [CrossRef] [PubMed]
6. Awadasseid, A.; Wu, Y.; Tanaka, Y.; Zhang, W. Current advances in the development of SARS-CoV-2 vaccines. *Int. J. Biol. Sci.* **2021**, *17*, 8–19. [CrossRef]
7. Chakraborty, S.; Mallajosyula, V.; Tato, C.M.; Tan, G.S.; Wang, T.T. SARS-CoV-2 vaccines in advanced clinical trials: Where do we stand? *Adv. Drug Deliv. Rev.* **2021**, *172*, 314–338. [CrossRef]
8. Logunov, D.Y.; Dolzhikova, I.V.; Zubkova, O.V.; Tukhvatullin, A.I.; Shcheblyakov, D.V.; Dzharullaeva, A.S.; Grousova, D.M.; Erokhova, A.S.; Kovyrshina, A.V.; Botikov, A.G.; et al. Safety and immunogenicity of an rAd26 and rAd5 vector-based heterologous prime-boost COVID-19 vaccine in two formulations: Two open, non-randomised phase 1/2 studies from Russia. *Lancet* **2020**, *396*, 887–897. [CrossRef]
9. Andryukov, B.G.; Besednova, N.N. Older adults: Panoramic view on the COVID-19 vaccination. *AIMS Public Health* **2021**, *8*, 388–415. [CrossRef]
10. Burki, T.K. The Russian vaccine for COVID-19. *Lancet Respir. Med.* **2020**, *8*, e85–e86. [CrossRef]
11. Keech, C.; Albert, G.; Cho, I.; Robertson, A.; Reed, P.; Neal, S.; Plested, J.S.; Zhu, M.; Cloney-Clark, S.; Zhou, H.; et al. Phase 1–2 Trial of a SARS-CoV-2 Recombinant Spike Protein Nanoparticle Vaccine. *N. Engl. J. Med.* **2020**, *383*, 2320–2332. [CrossRef] [PubMed]
12. Dai, L.; Gao, G.F. Viral targets for vaccines against COVID-19. *Nat. Rev. Immunol.* **2021**, *21*, 73–82. [CrossRef] [PubMed]
13. Al-Kassmy, J.; Pedersen, J.; Kobinger, G. Vaccine Candidates against Coronavirus Infections. Where Does COVID-19 Stand? *Viruses* **2020**, *12*, 861. [CrossRef]
14. Locht, C. Vaccines against COVID-19. *Anaesth. Crit. Care Pain Med.* **2020**, *39*, 703–705. [CrossRef] [PubMed]
15. Calina, D.; Docea, A.O.; Petrakis, D.; Egorov, A.M.; Ishmukhametov, A.A.; Gabibov, A.G.; Shtilman, M.I.; Kostoff, R.; Carvalho, F.; Vinceti, M.; et al. Towards effective COVID-19 vaccines: Updates, perspectives and challenges (Review). *Int. J. Mol. Med.* **2020**, *46*, 3–16. [CrossRef]
16. Kozlovskaya, L.I.; Piniaeva, A.N.; Ignatyev, G.M.; Gordeychuk, I.V.; Volok, V.P.; Rogova, Y.V.; Shishova, A.A.; Kovpak, A.A.; Ivin, Y.Y.; Antonova, L.P.; et al. Long-term humoral immunogenicity, safety and protective efficacy of inactivated vaccine against COVID-19 (CoviVac) in preclinical studies. *Emerg. Microbes Infect.* **2021**, *10*, 1790–1806. [CrossRef]
17. Baraniuk, C. COVID-19: What do we know about Sputnik V and other Russian vaccines? *BMJ* **2021**, *372*, n743. [CrossRef]
18. Asdaq, S.M.B.; Jomah, S.; Rabbani, S.I.; Alamri, A.M.; Alshammari, S.K.S.; Duwaidi, B.S.; Alshammari, M.S.; Alamri, A.S.; Alsanie, W.F.; Alhomrani, M.; et al. Insight into the Advances in Clinical Trials of SARS-CoV-2 Vaccines. *Can. J. Infect. Dis. Med. Microbiol.* **2022**, *2022*, 1–16. [CrossRef]
19. Hassine, I.H. COVID-19 vaccines and variants of concern: A review. *Rev. Med. Virol.* **2022**, *32*, e2313. [CrossRef]
20. Matveeva, O.; Ershov, A. Retrospective Cohort Study of the Effectiveness of the Sputnik V and EpiVacCorona Vaccines against the SARS-CoV-2 Delta Variant in Moscow (June–July 2021). *Vaccines* **2022**, *10*, 984. [CrossRef]
21. Tukhvatulin, A.I.; Dolzhikova, I.V.; Shcheblyakov, D.V.; Zubkova, O.V.; Dzharullaeva, A.S.; Kovyrshina, A.V.; Lubenets, N.L.; Grousova, D.M.; Erokhova, A.S.; Botikov, A.G.; et al. An open, non-randomised, phase 1/2 trial on the safety, tolerability, and immunogenicity of single-dose vaccine "Sputnik Light" for prevention of coronavirus infection in healthy adults. *Lancet Reg. Health Eur.* **2021**, *11*, 100241. [CrossRef] [PubMed]
22. Komissarov, A.A.; Dolzhikova, I.V.; Efimov, G.A.; Logunov, D.Y.; Mityaeva, O.; Molodtsov, I.A.; Naigovzina, N.B.; Peshkova, I.O.; Shcheblyakov, D.V.; Volchkov, P.; et al. Boosting of the SARS-CoV-2–Specific Immune Response after Vaccination with Single-Dose Sputnik Light Vaccine. *J. Immunol.* **2022**, *208*, 1139–1145. [CrossRef] [PubMed]
23. Vanaparthy, R.; Mohan, G.; Vasireddy, D.; Atluri, P. Review of COVID-19 viral vector-based vaccines and COVID-19 variants. *Infez. Med.* **2021**, *29*, 328–338. [CrossRef]
24. Ryzhikov, A.B.; Ryzhikov, E.A.; Bogryantseva, M.P.; Danilenko, E.D.; Imatdinov, I.R.; Nechaeva, E.A.; Pyankov, O.V.; Pyankova, O.G.; Susloparov, I.M.; Taranov, O.S.; et al. Immunogenicity and protectivity of the peptide candidate vaccine against SARS-CoV-2. *Ann. Russ. Acad. Med. Sci.* **2021**, *76*, 5–19. [CrossRef]

25. Ryzhikov, A.B.; Ryzhikov, E.A.; Bogryantseva, M.P.; Usova, S.V.; Danilenko, E.D.; Nechaeva, E.A.; Pyankov, O.V.; Pyankova, O.G.; Gudymo, A.S.; Bodnev, S.A.; et al. A single blind, placebo-controlled randomized study of the safety, reactogenicity and immunogenicity of the "EpiVacCorona" Vaccine for the prevention of COVID-19, in volunteers aged 18–60 years (phase I–II). *Russ. J. Infect. Immun.* **2021**, *11*, 283–296. [CrossRef]
26. Szmyd, B.; Bartoszek, A.; Karuga, F.F.; Staniecka, K.; Błaszczyk, M.; Radek, M. Medical Students and SARS-CoV-2 Vaccination: Attitude and Behaviors. *Vaccines* **2021**, *9*, 128. [CrossRef] [PubMed]
27. Lucia, V.C.; Kelekar, A.; Afonso, N.M. COVID-19 vaccine hesitancy among medical students. *J. Public Health* **2021**, *43*, 445–449. [CrossRef]
28. Saied, S.M.; Saied, E.M.; Kabbash, I.A.; Abdo, S.A.E. Vaccine hesitancy: Beliefs and barriers associated with COVID-19 vaccination among Egyptian medical students. *J. Med. Virol.* **2021**, *93*, 4280–4291. [CrossRef]
29. Albrecht, D. Vaccination, politics and COVID-19 impacts. *BMC Public Health* **2022**, *22*, 96. [CrossRef]
30. Faul, F.; Erdfelder, E.; Lang, A.-G.; Buchner, A. G*Power 3: A flexible statistical power analysis program for the social, behavioral, and biomedical sciences. *Behav. Res. Methods* **2007**, *39*, 175–191. [CrossRef]
31. Barello, S.; Nania, T.; Dellafiore, F.; Graffigna, G.; Caruso, R. 'Vaccine hesitancy' among university students in Italy during the COVID-19 pandemic. *Eur. J. Epidemiol.* **2020**, *35*, 781–783. [CrossRef] [PubMed]
32. Betsch, C.; Wicker, S. E-health use, vaccination knowledge and perception of own risk: Drivers of vaccination uptake in medical students. *Vaccine* **2012**, *30*, 1143–1148. [CrossRef] [PubMed]
33. Katz, M.; Azrad, M.; Glikman, D.; Peretz, A. COVID-19 Vaccination Compliance and Associated Factors among Medical Students during an Early Phase of Vaccination Rollout—A Survey from Israel. *Vaccines* **2021**, *10*, 27. [CrossRef] [PubMed]
34. Bălan, A.; Bejan, I.; Bonciu, S.; Eni, C.; Ruță, S. Romanian Medical Students' Attitude towards and Perceived Knowledge on COVID-19 Vaccination. *Vaccines* **2021**, *9*, 854. [CrossRef]
35. Harapan, H.; Wagner, A.L.; Yufika, A.; Winardi, W.; Anwar, S.; Gan, A.K.; Setiawan, A.M.; Rajamoorthy, Y.; Sofyan, H.; Mudatsir, M. Acceptance of a COVID-19 Vaccine in Southeast Asia: A Cross-Sectional Study in Indonesia. *Front. Public Health* **2020**, *8*, 381. [CrossRef]
36. Jain, J.; Saurabh, S.; Kumar, P.; Verma, M.K.; Goel, A.D.; Gupta, M.K.; Bhardwaj, P.; Raghav, P.R. COVID-19 vaccine hesitancy among medical students in India. *Epidemiol. Infect.* **2021**, *149*, e132. [CrossRef]
37. Kelekar, A.K.; Lucia, V.C.; Afonso, N.M.; Mascarenhas, A.K. COVID-19 vaccine acceptance and hesitancy among dental and medical students. *J. Am. Dent. Assoc.* **2021**, *152*, 596–603. [CrossRef]
38. Aragão, M.G.B.; Gomes, F.I.F.; Paixão-De-Melo, L.P.M.; Corona, S.A.M. Brazilian dental students and COVID-19: A survey on knowledge and perceptions. *Eur. J. Dent. Educ.* **2022**, *26*, 93–105. [CrossRef]
39. Qin, S.; Zhou, M.; Ding, Y. Risk Perception Measurement and Influencing Factors of COVID-19 in Medical College Students. *Front. Public Health* **2021**, *9*, 774572. [CrossRef]
40. Zhou, Y.; Wang, Y.; Li, Z. Intention to get vaccinated against COVID-19 among nursing students: A cross-sectional survey. *Nurse Educ. Today* **2021**, *107*, 105152. [CrossRef]
41. Ulbrichtova, R.; Svihrova, V.; Svihra, J. Prevalence of COVID-19 Vaccination among Medical Students: A Systematic Review and Meta-Analysis. *Int. J. Environ. Res. Public Health* **2022**, *19*, 4072. [CrossRef] [PubMed]
42. Sankova, M.V.; Kytko, O.V.; Vasil'Ev, Y.L.; Aleshkina, O.Y.; Diachkova, E.Y.; Darawsheh, H.M.; Kolsanov, A.V.; Dydykin, S.S. Medical Students' Reactive Anxiety as a Quality Criterion for Distance Learning during the SARS-COV-2 Pandemic. *Emerg. Sci. J.* **2021**, *5*, 86–93. [CrossRef]

International Journal of
Environmental Research and Public Health

MDPI

Article

The Impact of COVID-19 on Dental Treatment in Kuwait—A Retrospective Analysis from the Nation's Largest Hospital

Wasmiya Ali AlHayyan [1], Khalaf AlShammari [2], Falah AlAjmi [1] and Sharat Chandra Pani [3,*]

1 Al Jahra Specialist Center, Al Jahra, Kuwait; dr_ali@hotmail.com (W.A.A.); falahalajmi@gmail.com (F.A.)
2 Faculty of Dentistry, Kuwait Institution for Medical Specialization, Kuwait City, Kuwait; kalsham71@gmail.com
3 Schulich School of Medicine and Dentistry, University of Western Ontario, London, ON N6A 3K7, Canada
* Correspondence: spani@uwo.ca

Abstract: Background: The COVID-19 pandemic has changed the way dentistry has been practiced the world over. This study sought to assess the impact of the COVID-19 pandemic on the patterns of attendance for dental treatment in a large hospital in Kuwait through comparisons with data from the year prior to the pandemic. Methods: A total of 176,690 appointment records from 34,250 patients presenting to the AlJahra specialist hospital in Kuwait for dental treatment from April 2019 to March 2021 were analyzed. The types of procedures and the departments in which they presented were analyzed, and the patterns of attendance before and during the pandemic were compared. Results: While there was a significant reduction in the number of orthodontic, endodontic, and periodontal procedures, there were no impacts on oral surgery, restorative procedures, or pediatric dentistry. Conclusions: There has been a return in the number of patients obtaining dental treatment; however, there has been a definite shift in the use of certain dental procedures.

Keywords: access to dental care; COVID-19; dental public health

Citation: AlHayyan, W.A.; AlShammari, K.; AlAjmi, F.; Pani, S.C. The Impact of COVID-19 on Dental Treatment in Kuwait—A Retrospective Analysis from the Nation's Largest Hospital. *Int. J. Environ. Res. Public Health* **2022**, *19*, 9275. https://doi.org/10.3390/ijerph19159275

Academic Editor: Giuseppe Alessandro Scardina

Received: 7 June 2022
Accepted: 27 July 2022
Published: 29 July 2022

1. Introduction

The World Health Organization (WHO) announced the outbreak of a public health emergency of international concern on 30 January 2020, and a pandemic on 11 March 2020, affecting more than 7 million people in more than 188 countries [1]. The COVID-19 pandemic has changed the way dentistry has been practiced the world over [1–4]. The spread of the virus by aerosols has meant that dental practices the world over have had to find ways to contain aerosols in practices [5]. There is also data emerging showing that the pandemic has had different impacts on different dental specialties [5–7].

The impact of COVID-19 in Kuwait has been documented in the literature and the State adopted aggressive measures toward the containment of the pandemic, including an early and aggressive lockdown between 1 April and 30 May 2020. Between the declaration of the pandemic in March 2020 and the first administration of vaccines in April–May 2021, Kuwait saw variations in both the number of cases and mortality from COVID-19 [8]. There is, however, no data on how these factors affected the attendance of patients in dental clinics in Kuwait.

Dental care in Kuwait has been provided to all residents using a combination of subsidies and benefits since 1951. However, since 1992, growth and improvements in the economy have meant that dental care in Kuwait is provided by both government hospitals and private dental clinics [9]. While private clinics provide services for a fee, the government hospital provides free dental care to all who are eligible. Despite the growth of private dental care in Kuwait, the role of government centers in the provision of dental care and their impact on the overall well-being of the people of Kuwait has been documented in the literature [9,10].

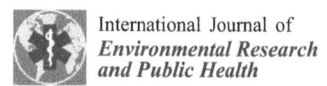

The Kuwait dental administration at the ministry of health in Kuwait has built an integrated medical system based on recommended scientific policies and a clear methodology in the different dental specialties representing the largest medical specialties with regard to finance and human resources. A total of 1,083,272 patients benefit from dental services provided in polyclinics at distinct residential areas in Kuwait. The AlJahra Specialized Dental Center (ASDC) is the largest of the different governmental polyclinics, serving nearly 22.1% of the patients referred from polyclinics to specialized centers [10].

The ASDC is part of the new AlJahra hospital in the AlJahra governate, the largest governate among the six Kuwaiti governates, with the highest population density [9]. The ASDC serves the AlJahra governate and the surrounding AlJahra districts, with a population of 452,596 people [3]. Prior to the pandemic, this was one of the largest dental treatment centers in Kuwait, seeing over 20,000 patients per year.

Data are emerging from around the world showing that the initial reluctance of individuals to seek dental treatment during the pandemic has been replaced by differing access to dental care [3,11–13]. While there have been some attempts to analyze data from multiple centers [14–16], there is little longitudinal data from a large public hospital. Newer variants of the virus and increased transmissibility mean the world has seen the pandemic slowly start to show features of an endemic. Data on how services were impacted by the COVID-19 pandemic are important for developing a better understanding of how dentists across the globe can deal with the challenges posed by this new phase of the disease. This study sought to assess the impact of the COVID-19 pandemic on patterns of attendance for dental treatment at the AlJahra Specialized Dental Center (ASDC) and compare them to data from the year prior to the pandemic.

2. Materials and Methods

2.1. Ethics Approval

Ethics approval for the study was obtained from the Standing Committee for the Co-ordination of Medical and Health Research, Ministry of Health, Government of Kuwait, to be carried out at AlJahra Hospital (1829/2021). All patients attending the hospital signed a form consenting to the use of their anonymized data for research purposes. The parents of children aged below 18 years signed this form on their behalf.

2.2. Data Collection

The data were collected retrospectively from the patient management system (Patient Statistic Program-Microsoft Access 2000, Microsoft Corp., Palo Alto, CA, USA). Data regarding the age, gender, and nationality of the patients, as well as the department providing the treatment, were collected. Monthly COVID-19 case rates and vaccination rates for the AlJahra governate were obtained from the Central Statistical Bureau. The codes for each department were entered before each visit and were included in the data mining for the current study. The details of the appointment, the number of visits for each procedure, and the time taken per appointment were not mined for the current study.

2.3. Data Analysis

Patient data were exported using Microsoft Excel (Microsoft Corp., Palo Alto, CA, USA) and analyzed using the SPSS version 25 data processing software (IBM-SPSS, Armonk, NY, USA). Descriptive data were tabulated and the significance levels of differences among gender and nationality were calculated. Differences between pre-pandemic and pandemic levels of attendance were compared according to specialty, with differences calculated using the binomial test. Differences between the genders in each department were measured separately before and during the pandemic and tested for significance using the binomial test. All tests were carried out with a level of significance of $p < 0.05$.

3. Results

The sample was comprised of 176,690 records of appointment registration data from 34,250 patients who presented to the dental clinics of AlJahra hospital from March 2019 to March 2021. The sample was divided into two main groups: records of patients visiting before the pandemic (April 2019–March 2020) and during the pandemic (April 2020–March 2021) (Figure 1). Overall, there were fewer appointments during the pandemic (n = 83,813) when compared to the previous year (n = 92,598). A description of the mined data is presented in Table 1.

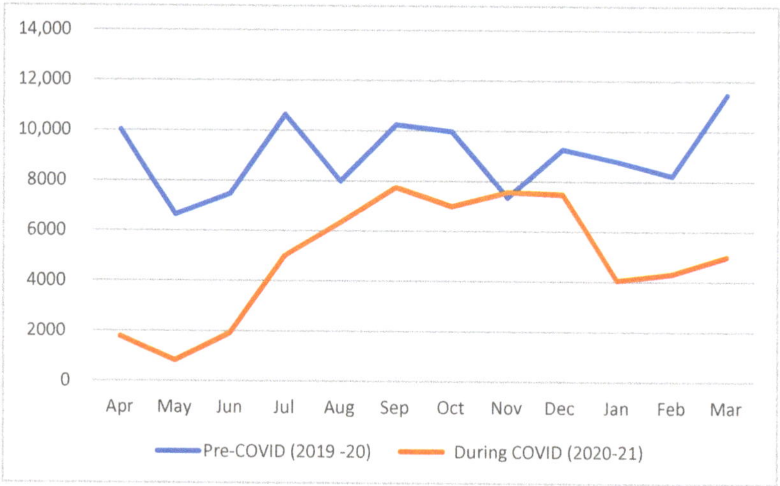

Figure 1. Impact of COVID-19 on overall patient presentation.

Table 1. Demographic profile of the population.

	Gender	Age Group			
		Below 12 Years	13–44 Years	45–64 Years	Above 65 Years
No. of Patients	Male	1123	8113	3101	883
	Female	1213	12,677	6234	906
No. of Appointments	Male	15,605	40,391	11,667	2219
	Female	16,784	69,027	18,583	2414

When divided according to gender, it was observed that there were significantly more female patients seen in all departments except for the COVID-19 unit and the pediatric dentistry department. This trend was the same before and during the pandemic (Table 2).

The impact of the pandemic was compared by specialty (Table 3). It was observed that different specialties were affected differently. While there was a significant reduction in patients seen in orthodontics, endodontics, and periodontics, no significant reductions were observed in prosthodontics. In both pediatric dentistry and oral surgery, there was an increase in the number of patients seen, although the differences were not statistically significant.

When the types of treatment rendered were tabulated (Figure 2), it was observed that all types of procedures were impacted by the first shutdown from April 2020 to June 2020. During this period, almost no aerosol-generating procedures were performed (Table 4). However, after the lifting of restrictions, a rebound in the number of procedures was observed (Figure 2). It was observed that variations were greatest among procedures such as prosthodontics, restorative procedures, and orthodontics (Figure 2).

Table 2. Attendance differences according to gender.

	Department	Gender				p *
		Male		Female		
		Count	Row N %	Count	Row N %	
During the Pandemic (2020–2021)	Pediatric Dentistry	7162	47.9%	7786	52.1%	0.187
	COVID-19 Unit	N/A	N/A	N/A	N/A	N/A
	Prosthodontics/Operative	5270	37.0%	8958	63.0%	<0.001 **
	Orthodontics	2717	30.2%	6270	69.8%	<0.001 **
	Oral Surgery	12,880	41.7%	18,032	58.3%	<0.001 **
	Endodontics	3831	38.2%	6204	61.8%	<0.001 **
	Periodontics	1645	35.0%	3054	65.0%	<0.001 **
Pre-Pandemic (2019–2020)	Pediatric Dentistry	7073	48.0%	7664	52.0%	0.865
	COVID-19 Unit	338	49.3%	347	50.7%	0.906
	Prosthodontics/Operative	5026	33.4%	10,030	66.6%	<0.001 **
	Orthodontics	3576	33.7%	7027	66.3%	<0.001 **
	Oral Surgery	11,253	40.5%	16,519	59.5%	<0.001 **
	Endodontics	6247	37.9%	10,253	62.1%	<0.001 **
	Periodontics	2659	36.7%	4585	63.3%	<0.001 **

* Calculated using the binomial test. ** Differences significant at $p < 0.05$.

Table 3. Impact of the pandemic on attendance by specialty.

	During the Pandemic (2020–2021)	Pre-Pandemic (2019–2020)	p *
Pediatric Dentistry	14,948	14,737	0.564
COVID-19 Unit	NA	685	NA
Prosthodontic/Operative	14,228	15,056	0.148
Orthodontics	8987	10,603	0.021 **
Oral Surgery	30,912	27,772	0.076
Endodontics	10,035	16,500	0.005 **
Periodontics	4699	7244	0.001 **

* Calculated using the binomial test. ** Differences significant at $p < 0.05$.

Table 4. Type of procedure performed by month from March 2019 to March 2021.

	Examination	Restorative	Pulp Therapy/ Endodontics	Surgery	Adjustment of Orthodontic Bracket and Appliance	Impression, Tooth Preparation, Crown Cementation	Implant, Scaling, and Root Planning
Mar-19	2547	589	1149	3621	288	1075	151
Apr-19	2484	618	1712	3175	378	1130	379
May-19	1450	397	771	2511	371	799	163
Jun-19	2827	318	686	2402	345	555	226
Jul-19	4313	524	859	3172	128	1180	265
Aug-19	3543	490	820	2248	210	399	195
Sep-19	4694	556	1170	2295	408	748	205
Oct-19	4025	440	953	2748	635	727	218
Nov-19	3035	374	768	1634	477	660	188
Dec-19	3431	477	925	2670	582	670	235
Jan-20	2090	399	697	3502	378	1216	365
Feb-20	2073	620	1712	2155	371	796	305
Mar-20	3574	706	1358	3409	309	1441	181
Apr-20	1137	4	5	550	0	35	0
May-20	397	0	0	426	0	1	0
Jun-20	1088	28	38	747	0	0	0
Jul-20	1777	349	591	1208	170	550	19
Aug-20	2128	531	862	1435	231	592	77
Sep-20	2292	651	970	1475	197	1484	102
Oct-20	2151	481	755	1366	448	1417	83
Nov-20	1981	503	849	1506	225	1912	139
Dec-20	2098	495	826	1683	195	1478	120
Jan-21	2251	238	614	1693	640	500	152
Feb-21	2338	287	1067	1481	570	426	146
Mar-21	2406	337	680	2024	627	721	195

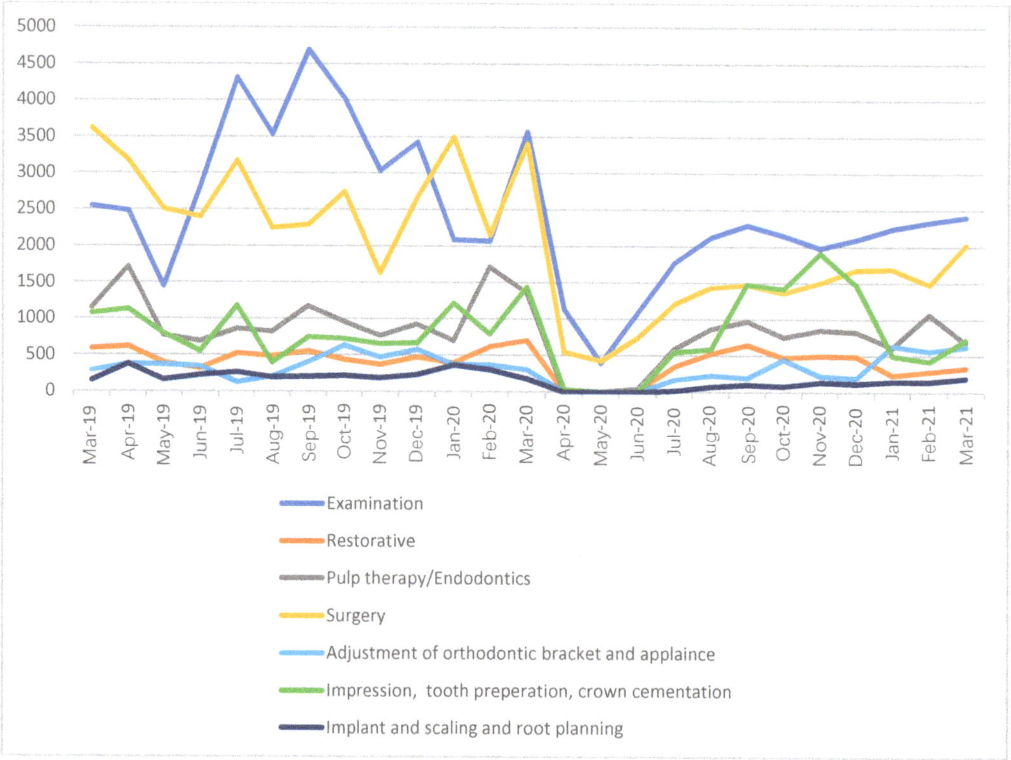

Figure 2. The number of treatments rendered before and during the pandemic, by type of treatment.

4. Discussion

It has now been over two years since the first COVID-19 case was diagnosed, and the impacts on dentistry are becoming clearer [14,15,17,18]. This study aimed to follow the patterns of patient care over a one-year period from the implementation of the first COVID-19 restrictions in Kuwait. As data emerge on the ways that dental practices are adapting to pandemic-induced restrictions globally, this study sought to visualize the changing patterns in a large governmental hospital as the pandemic progressed.

The initial stages of the pandemic, from April 2020 to July 2020, were periods of effective shutdown for dental practices across the globe [8]. The lack of clear guidelines on the risks of aerosols, combined with global shutdowns and/or lockdowns, meant that elective dental procedures were not performed [4,18,19]; this is reflected in the drop in cases seen between April and July 2020. As restrictions on aerosol-generating procedures were gradually lifted, there was a slow increase in the number of patients seen. Our data show that between June and July 2020 there was a sharp increase in the number of patients seen for examination and surgery. This is explained by the fact that as operatories were allowed to perform aerosol-generating procedures, emergency procedures were re-prioritized. This is also in keeping with studies that showed that emergency procedures in the early days of the pandemic were restricted to extractions [4,17].

The increase in restorative and endodontic procedures during the period from July 2020 to the end of the study is of great significance. Our data suggest that there was a gradual increase in the number of these procedures being performed. The data also show that once these procedures were being performed, there was little variation in the number of procedures. This suggests that endodontic and restorative procedures are essential to the well-being of individuals. The tendency to restrict emergency procedures to extractions in the early days of the pandemic was based largely on the fact that there were insufficient operatories to manage aerosol-generating procedures [4,19,20]. The pandemic has resulted in the re-designing of dental operatories, both in small practices and large hospitals [2,3,5,19,21]. The data from this study show that the availability of sufficient rooms to perform these procedures is essential for the delivery of optimal dental care. The data also show that the hospital was able to create an infrastructure that could support the practice of aerosol-generating procedures. In this case, the hospital was a public organization, and funding from the government allowed for the creation of the necessary infrastructure. The financial toll on practices both large and small is beyond the scope of the current paper but is an important area for further research.

The fact that there were variations in orthodontic procedures suggests that these procedures are perhaps viewed as non-essential. While an argument can be made for these procedures to be provided a lower priority than pain-relieving procedures, such as endodontics, the impacts of treatment suspension on the outcomes of tertiary dental care are emerging [22,23]. Literature shows that prolonging or postponing orthodontic care that has already started can result in care being extended for long periods, with adverse outcomes, not only for orthodontic outcomes but also for oral hygiene [24].

The current dataset used secondary data, and since the operatory used for the provision of ultrasonic scaling is the same as the operatory used for the placement of implants, the data on the numbers of these procedures are presented together. The results are worrisome, as they show a significantly lower number of procedures when compared to restorative or endodontic care. Good ultrasonic scaling has long been viewed as the bedrock of dental hygiene maintenance [7]. However, the restrictions imposed on aerosol-generating procedures, have meant that, across the world, dentists have had to either limit or altogether stop the number of ultrasonic scaling procedures [5,7,14,15,18]. The results of the current study show that while the rates of endodontic and restorative procedures classified as "essential" have returned to pre-pandemic levels, the rates of scaling/root-planing/implant procedures are at half the pre-pandemic levels.

Since the pandemic began, research has focused on both minimizing aerosols in dental practices and the optimal allocation of rooms where aerosol-generating procedures can be safely carried out [15–17]. The results of this study highlight the fact that pain-relieving procedures, such as restorative care, oral surgery, and endodontics quickly bounced back to pre-pandemic levels. A more interesting find is that while the placement of orthodontic brackets had returned to pre-pandemic levels by March 2021, ultrasonic scaling procedures had not. This finding mirrors global trends that show that while non-aerosol generating procedures quickly return to pre-pandemic levels, practices (both large and small) struggle to create new infrastructure to cope with the requirements for aerosol-generating procedures [12,17]. Orthodontic care is known to be associated with poorer oral hygiene outcomes [21]. The absence of or limitations in access to good ultrasonic scaling can have potential adverse effects that need to be addressed.

The results of this study have to be viewed keeping in mind the overall changes in dentistry, both globally and within the Middle Eastern region [25,26]. The results of this study are in keeping with those of Cha and Cohen, who showed that there were significantly fewer adults who received a dental check-up in 2019 compared to 2020 [25]. The practice of dentistry in large hospital-based or hospital-like situations differs in many ways from the practice in a smaller individual or group dental practice. Since the beginning of the pandemic, there have been several factors that have affected the practice of dentistry in hospital settings. The fact that the pattern of practices changed during the pandemic has been previously documented. However, our results suggest that even after the lifting of restrictions there are certain shifts in the practice of dentistry that have continued to remain in place. This is in keeping with other hospital data from the region, which suggested changes in dental practice in a hospital setting in Saudi Arabia [27]. It is, therefore, reasonable to assume that large hospitals in the region will need to further evaluate the impact these changes have on the cost of care, the efficiency of care delivery, and the impact of these changes on patient satisfaction.

There are certain limitations of this study. The study only looked at practices in a hospital setting and does not reflect the challenges faced by smaller practices. Furthermore, the scope of the current study was only the overall pattern of attendance of the patients. The actual treatment rendered and the number of appointments per procedure were not recorded and were beyond the scope of this study. Despite these limitations, the study has many strengths, including the large sample size and the fact that the study followed the population into 2021 to fully visualize the longer-term impacts of COVID-19-related changes on the practice of dentistry.

5. Conclusions

The results of this study show that while attendance in dental clinics at the AlJahra hospital has nearly returned to pre-pandemic levels, there have been significant shifts in the types of procedures performed. The long-term impacts of these shifts are deserving of future research in order to provide comprehensive dental care to patients as well as to better plan for future waves of the pandemic.

Author Contributions: Conceptualization, W.A.A. and S.C.P.; methodology, S.C.P.; software, W.A.A. and S.C.P.; validation, K.A. and F.A.; formal analysis, S.C.P.; investigation, W.A.A.; resources, W.A.A., K.A. and F.A.; data curation, W.A.A.; writing—original draft preparation, S.C.P.; writing—review and editing, W.A.A. and K.A. All authors have read and agreed to the published version of the manuscript.

Funding: The APC was funded by the Ministry of Health, Government of Kuwait.

Institutional Review Board Statement: The study was conducted in accordance with the Declaration of Helsinki, and approved by the Institutional Review Board (or Ethics Committee) of the Standing Committee for the Co-ordination of Medical and Health Research, of the AlJahra Hospital (1829/2021). Ministry of Health, Government of Kuwait.

Informed Consent Statement: All patients attending the hospital sign a form consenting to the use of anonymized data for research purposes.

Data Availability Statement: Data will be made available upon reasonable request to the authors.

Conflicts of Interest: The authors declare no conflict of interest.

References

1. Campus, G.; Diaz Betancourt, M.; Cagetti, M.G.; Giacaman, R.A.; Manton, D.J.; Douglas, G.; Carvalho, T.S.; Carvalho, J.C.; Vukovic, A.; Cortés-Martinicorena, F.J.; et al. The COVID-19 pandemic and its global effects on dental practice. An international survey. *J. Dent.* **2021**, *114*, 103749. [CrossRef] [PubMed]
2. Farshidfar, N.; Jafarpour, D.; Hamedani, S.; Dziedzic, A.; Tanasiewicz, M. Proposal for Tier-Based Resumption of Dental Practice Determined by COVID-19 Rate, Testing and COVID-19 Vaccination: A Narrative Perspective. *J. Clin. Med.* **2021**, *10*, 2116. [CrossRef] [PubMed]
3. Dong, Q.; Kuria, A.; Weng, Y.; Liu, Y.; Cao, Y. Impacts of the COVID-19 epidemic on the department of stomatology in a tertiary hospital: A case study in the General Hospital of the Central Theater Command, Wuhan, China. Community Dent. *Oral Epidemiol.* **2021**, *49*, 557–564. [CrossRef] [PubMed]
4. Salgarello, S.; Salvadori, M.; Mazzoleni, F.; Francinelli, J.; Bertoletti, P.; Audino, E.; Garo, M.L. The New Normalcy in Dentistry after the COVID-19 Pandemic: An Italian Cross-Sectional Survey. *Dent. J.* **2021**, *9*, 86. [CrossRef]
5. Singh, H.; Maurya, R.K.; Sharma, P.; Kapoor, P.; Mittal, T. Aerosol generating procedural risks and concomitant mitigation strategies in orthodontics amid COVID-19 pandemic—An updated evidence-based review. *Int. Orthod.* **2021**, *19*, 329–345. [CrossRef]
6. El-Boghdadly, K.; Cook, T.M.; Goodacre, T.; Kua, J.; Blake, L.; Denmark, S.; McNally, S.; Mercer, N.; Moonesinghe, S.R.; Summerton, D.J. SARS-CoV-2 infection, COVID-19 and timing of elective surgery: A multidisciplinary consensus statement on behalf of the Association of Anaesthetists, the Centre for Peri-operative Care, the Federation of Surgical Specialty Associations, the Royal College. *Anaesthesia* **2021**, *76*, 940–946. [CrossRef]
7. Pierre-Bez, A.C.; Agostini-Walesch, G.M.; Bradford Smith, P.; Hong, Q.; Hancock, D.S.; Davis, M.; Marcelli-Munk, G.; Mitchell, J.C. Ultrasonic scaling in COVID-era dentistry: A quantitative assessment of aerosol spread during simulated and clinical ultrasonic scaling procedures. *Int. J. Dent. Hyg.* **2021**, *19*, 474–480. [CrossRef]

8. Alkhamis, M.A.; Al Youha, S.; Khajah, M.M.; Haider, N.B.; Alhardan, S.; Nabeel, A.; Al Mazeedi, S.; Al-Sabah, S.K. Spatiotemporal dynamics of the COVID-19 pandemic in the State of Kuwait. *Int. J. Infect. Dis.* **2020**, *98*, 153–160. [CrossRef]
9. Al-Mudaf, B.A.; Moussa, M.A.A.; Al-Terky, M.A.; Al-Dakhil, G.D.; El-Farargy, A.E.; Al-Ouzairi, S.S. Patient satisfaction with three dental speciality services: A centre-based study. *Med. Princ. Pract.* **2003**, *12*, 39–43. [CrossRef]
10. Alhashem, A.M.; Alquraini, H.; Chowdhury, R.I. Factors influencing patient satisfaction in primary healthcare clinics in Kuwait. *Int. J. Health Care Qual. Assur.* **2011**, *24*, 249–262. [CrossRef]
11. Amato, A.; Ciacci, C.; Martina, S.; Caggiano, M.; Amato, M. COVID-19: The Dentists' Perceived Impact on the Dental Practice. *Eur. J. Dent.* **2021**, *15*, 469–474. [CrossRef]
12. Rehman, R.; Jawed, S.; Ali, R.; Noreen, K.; Baig, M.; Baig, J. COVID-19 Pandemic Awareness, Attitudes, and Practices Among the Pakistani General Public. *Front. Public Health* **2021**, *9*, 588537. [CrossRef]
13. Alkhalifah, F.N.; Tobbal, A.Y.; Fried, J.L. COVID-19 impact, knowledge and preparedness among dental hygienists in Saudi Arabia: A cross-sectional study. *Int. J. Dent. Hyg.* **2021**, *19*, 464–473. [CrossRef]
14. Ali, S. Dental practice during the era of COVID-19 pandemic: An Egyptian experience. *Oral Dis.* **2021**. [CrossRef]
15. Ostrc, T.; Pavlović, K.; Fidler, A. Urgent dental care on a national level during the COVID-19 epidemic. *Clin. Exp. Dent. Res.* **2021**, *7*, 271–278. [CrossRef]
16. Abdulkareem, A.A.; Abdulbaqi, H.R.; Alshami, M.L.; Al-Rawi, N.H. Oral health awareness, attitude towards dental treatment, fear of infection and economic impact during COVID-19 pandemic in the Middle East. *Int. J. Dent. Hyg.* **2021**, *19*, 295–304. [CrossRef]
17. Iurcov, R.; Pop, L.M.; Ciavoi, G.; Iorga, M. Evaluating the Practice of Preventive Behaviors and the Fear of COVID-19 among Dentists in Oradea Metropolitan Area after the First Wave of Pandemic; a Cross-Sectional Study. *Healthcare* **2021**, *9*, 443. [CrossRef]
18. Pietrzak, P.; Hanke, W. COVID-19 and dentistry-safety issues regarding doctor and patient situation in time of vaccine availability. *Med. Pract.* **2021**, *72*, 729–737. [CrossRef]
19. Vernon, J.J.; Black, E.V.I.; Dennis, T.; Devine, D.A.; Fletcher, L.; Wood, D.J.; Nattress, B.R. Dental Mitigation Strategies to Reduce Aerosolization of SARS-CoV-2. *J. Dent. Res.* **2021**, *100*, 1461–1467. [CrossRef]
20. Aravind, A.; Nair, S.; Aparna, T.K.; Thomas, A.J.; Oommen, S.; Vijayan, A. Attention to COVID-19 Pandemic among Dental Experts of Kerala State, India: A Knowledge, Attitude, and Practice Study. *J. Pharm. Bioallied Sci.* **2021**, *13*, S836–S840. [CrossRef]
21. Melo, P.; Barbosa, J.M.; Jardim, L.; Carrilho, E.; Portugal, J. COVID-19 Management in Clinical Dental Care. Part I: Epidemiology, Public Health Implications, and Risk Assessment. *Int. Dent. J.* **2021**, *71*, 251–262. [CrossRef] [PubMed]
22. Martina, S.; Amato, A.; Faccioni, P.; Iandolo, A.; Amato, M.; Rongo, R. The perception of COVID-19 among Italian dental patients: An orthodontic point of view. *Prog. Orthod.* **2021**, *22*, 11. [CrossRef] [PubMed]
23. Umeh, O.D.; Utomi, I.L.; Isiekwe, I.G.; Aladenika, E.T. Impact of the coronavirus disease 2019 pandemic on orthodontic patients and their attitude to orthodontic treatment. *Am. J. Orthod. Dentofac. Orthop.* **2021**, *159*, e399–e409. [CrossRef] [PubMed]
24. Quan, S.; Guo, Y.; Zhou, J.; Zhang, G.; Xing, K.; Mei, H.; Li, J. Orthodontic emergencies and mental state of Chinese orthodontic patients during the COVID-19 pandemic. *BMC Oral Health* **2021**, *21*, 477. [CrossRef]
25. Alamoudi, R.A.; Basudan, S.; Mahboub, M.; Baghlaf, K. Impact of COVID-19 Pandemic on Dental Treatment in Children: A Retrospective Cross-Sectional Analysis in Jeddah City. *Clin. Cosmet. Investig. Dent.* **2022**, *14*, 95–102. [CrossRef]
26. Cha, A.E.; Cohen, R.A. Dental Care Utilization Among Adults Aged 18–64: United States, 2019 and 2020. *NCHS Data Brief* **2022**, *435*, 1–8.
27. Alassaf, A.; Almulhim, B.; Alghamdi, S.A.; Mallineni, S.K. Perceptions and Preventive Practices Regarding COVID-19 Pandemic Outbreak and Oral Health Care Perceptions during the Lockdown: A Cross-Sectional Survey from Saudi Arabia. *Healthcare* **2021**, *9*, 959. [CrossRef]

International Journal of
Environmental Research and Public Health

MDPI

Article

Dental Care and Education Facing Highly Transmissible SARS-CoV-2 Variants: Prospective Biosafety Setting: Prospective, Single-Arm, Single-Center Study

Andrej Thurzo [1,*], Wanda Urbanová [2], Iveta Waczulíková [3], Veronika Kurilová [4], Bela Mriňáková [5], Helena Kosnáčová [6,7], Branislav Gális [8], Ivan Varga [9], Marek Matajs [1] and Bohuslav Novák [1,*]

1 Department of Stomatology and Maxillofacial Surgery, Faculty of Medicine, Comenius University in Bratislava, 81250 Bratislava, Slovakia; marek.matajs@fmed.uniba.sk
2 Department of Orthodontics and Cleft Anomalies, Dental Clinic 3rd Medical Faculty Charles University, Faculty Hospital Kralovske Vinohrady, 10034 Prague, Czech Republic; wanda.urbanova@gmail.com
3 Department of Nuclear Physics and Biophysics, Faculty of Mathematics, Physics and Informatics, Comenius University, Mlynska dolina F1, 84248 Bratislava, Slovakia; iveta.waczulikova@fmph.uniba.sk
4 Faculty of Electrical Engineering and Information Technology, Slovak University of Technology, Ilkovicova 3, 81219 Bratislava, Slovakia; veronika.hanuskova@gmail.com
5 1st Department of Oncology, Medical Faculty, Comenius University, St. Elisabeth Cancer Institute, 81250 Bratislava, Slovakia; bela.mrinakova@ousa.sk
6 Department of Simulation and Virtual Medical Education, Faculty of Medicine, Comenius University in Bratislava, Sasinkova 4, 81272 Bratislava, Slovakia; helena.svobodova@fmed.uniba.sk
7 Department of Genetics, Cancer Research Institute, Biomedical Research Center, Slovak Academy Sciences, Dúbravská Cesta 9, 84505 Bratislava, Slovakia
8 Department of Oral and Maxillofacial Surgery, Medical Faculty, Comenius University, University Hospital Bratislava, 81499 Bratislava, Slovakia; brano.galis@gmail.com
9 Institute of Histology and Embryology, Faculty of Medicine, Comenius University in Bratislava, 81372 Bratislava, Slovakia; ivan.varga@fmed.uniba.sk
* Correspondence: thurzo3@uniba.sk (A.T.); bohuslav.novak@fmed.uniba.sk (B.N.); Tel.: +421-903-110-107 (A.T.)

Citation: Thurzo, A.; Urbanová, W.; Waczulíková, I.; Kurilová, V.; Mriňáková, B.; Kosnáčová, H.; Gális, B.; Varga, I.; Matajs, M.; Novák, B. Dental Care and Education Facing Highly Transmissible SARS-CoV-2 Variants: Prospective Biosafety Setting: Prospective, Single-Arm, Single-Center Study. *Int. J. Environ. Res. Public Health* **2022**, *19*, 7693. https://doi.org/10.3390/ijerph19137693

Academic Editors: Giuseppe Alessandro Scardina and Paul B. Tchounwou

Received: 19 May 2022
Accepted: 21 June 2022
Published: 23 June 2022

Abstract: With the arrival of the highly transmissible Omicron variants (BA.4 and BA.5), dentistry faces another seasonal challenge to preserve the biosafety of dental care and education. With the aim of protecting patients, students, teachers and healthcare professionals, this paper introduces a prospective sustainable biosafety setting for everyday dental care and education. The setting developed by dental clinicians, epidemiologists, and teachers of dentistry consists of a combination of modern technologies focused on the air-borne part of the viral pathway. The introduced biosafety setting has been clinically evaluated after 18 months of application in the real clinical environment. The protocol has three fundamental pillars: (1) UVC air disinfection; (2) air saturation with certified virucidal essences with nebulizing diffusers; (3) complementary solutions including telehealth and 3D printing. A pseudonymous online smart form was used as the evaluation method. The protocol operates on the premise that everybody is a hypothetical asymptomatic carrier. The results of a clinical evaluation of 115 patient feedbacks imply that no virus transmission from patient to patient or from doctor to nurse was observed or reported using this protocol, and vice versa, although nine patients retrospectively admitted that the clinic visit is likely to be infectious. Despite these promising results, a larger clinical sample and exposition to the current mutated strains are needed for reliable conclusions about protocol virucidal efficiency in current dental environments.

Keywords: dental education; biosafety; dentistry; orthodontics; sustainability; COVID-19; infection; prevention; teledentistry; UVC; virucidal oil dispersion

1. Introduction

Clinical dentistry as well as dental education experienced more than two difficult years of the SARS-CoV-2 pandemic. Initially, some experts expressed doubts about the potential of this new virus to cause a global pandemic with significant socio-economic impacts. This has also affected the domain of the dental community, including clinical care and education [1–8].

The world is now confronted with highly transmissible variants of SARS-CoV-2 (Omicron strains BA.1 overtaken by more transmissible BA.2) causing COVID-19, although these are fortunately less virulent than previous strains. Strains BA.4 and BA.5 are at our doorstep suggesting a possible autumn breakout. The dentistry sector is now facing these highly transmissible SARS-CoV-2 variants with currently highly protected, albeit waning, immunity in the population after mass vaccinations. There is a demand for a biosafe workflow in dental care and education. Even though COVID-19 is currently less lethal than ever before, the overall risk of infection, post-viral syndrome (long COVID-19) remains higher than at the beginning of the pandemic. So far, dental professionals have been able to anticipate the risks of incoming waves and their seasonality. Biosafety measures in dental offices have been repeatedly revised to protect patients and healthcare workers [2,9–16]. Dentists have changed their behavior and adapted their workflows [1,2,17].

Dental care and education are characterized by close personal contacts and treatment procedures that produce aerosols. Dental healthcare professionals, including dentists, dental assistants, dental hygienists, and nurses were aware of the high risk of exposure in the early stages of the COVID-19 pandemic [18,19]. The fact is that dentists are at a high risk of contracting COVID-19 from their patients because of its transmission by respiratory droplets and the use of dental handpieces that can generate aerosols [20,21], as well as the physical proximity of their patients [19,22,23]. Understanding the significance of aerosol transmission and its implications in dentistry can facilitate the identification and possible correction of negligence in daily dental practice [24]. The mitigation of particles that can carry the virus, and thus the mitigation of the risk of pathogen transmission in dental offices, often confirm the high effectiveness of personal protective equipment in protecting patients and dentists from aerosols [25].

Dental education struggling with the biosafety of students, patients and educators was characteristic, along with its high adaptability to implementing modern technologies, including online educational platforms, teledentistry diagnostics and various e-learning tools [8,26–28]. In 2021, Varvara et al., published a study designed to determine the undergraduate student perception of e-learning educational methods. The student feedback showed significant appreciation ($p < 0.05$) of the new methods, although a lack of practical training was significantly perceived as an important problem in the structure of their new curriculum [29].

In March 2020, nearly 200,000 dentists in the United States closed their offices to patients in fear, fueled by concerns that aerosols generated during dental procedures are potential vehicles for transmission of respiratory pathogens through saliva [30]. The findings published by Meethil et al., in the Journal of Dental Research [31] suggest lower risks for transmission of the SARS-CoV-2 virus during dental procedures than anticipated.

Preprocedural rinsing is one of the biosafety precautions introduced later in this work. The authors have learned from their clinical experience that this can occasionally lead to a patient developing cough, and therefore providing the exact opposite of the intended effect. While preprocedural rinsing has been encouraged since the onset of the pandemic, the guidelines on which antiviral to use were unclear. The American Dental Association (ADA) initially recommended 1.5% hydrogen peroxide and 0.2% povidone iodine for use as an antiviral prerinse [32,33]. When actual antiviral testing of these commercial rinses on SARS-CoV-2 finally became available, a different picture began to emerge. While the ADA recommended 1.5% hydrogen peroxide as an antiviral prerinse, the Centers for Disease Control and Prevention (CDC) advised that 1.5% hydrogen peroxide needs 18 to 20 min to inactivate rhinovirus, the virus that causes the common cold [34]. In October 2020, an extensive review inspecting the antiviral efficacy of hydrogen peroxide mouthwash was published in the Journal of Hospital Infection [35]. The authors concluded that: "there is no scientific evidence supporting the indication of hydrogen peroxide mouthwash for control of the viral load regarding SARS-CoV-2 or any other viruses in saliva." [35]. As a result of this knowledge and additional in vitro and in vivo tests, the Royal College of Dental Surgeons and the Canadian Dental Hygienists Association have advised all their constituents to discontinue the use of hydrogen peroxide as an antiviral prerinse [36]. In August 2020, the Antiviral Research Institute of Utah State University piloted a study of the antiviral efficacy of several oral rinses against SARS-CoV-2 [37]. Of all the rinses evaluated, 0.12% chlorhexidine gluconate and 1.5% hydrogen peroxide were inadequately effective, even after 60 s of exposure. While 0.2% povidone iodine performed slightly better, the only rinse that completely inactivated SARS-CoV-2 was a 100 ppm molecular iodine rinse. It was completely effective within 30 s. None of the iodine rinses were cytotoxic, but the hydrogen peroxide and chlorhexidine gluconate rinses were. At present, molecular iodine rinse is the clear evidence-based winner as a prerinse for SARS-CoV-2. This is particularly important considering that many other oral rinses are neutralized in the presence of saliva [38–43]. Oral rinses are a regular part of various dental biosafety protocols.

Dental care is often provided to oncological or other immunocompromised patients. It is crucial that precautionary measures are implemented so that these patients can be treated in a safe environment. A timely adaptation of clinical workflows and implementation of practice modification measures was observed throughout the world [15,44–47]. These, with the arrival of significantly more infectious Omicron-strains, need to be revised [45]. Moreover, dental care is essential in dealing with toxicity of anti-cancer treatments such as oral mucositis, xerostomia, trismus, osteoradionecrosis, and opportunistic infections [48]. Optimal safety protocols must be applied to minimize the risks in this population during dental care and education.

Current preventive biosafety measures often consider the possible specific intraoral manifestation of COVID-19. Triad xerostomia, taste and smell dysfunction, and oral mucosal lesions were identified as common manifestations with previous variants; however, with still controversial causality in omicron variants, xerostomia, taste, and smell dysfunctions are no longer common symptoms. A causal relationship between oral lesions and COVID-19 has been proven [49–53].

The pandemic has had a significant impact not only on dentists and their colleagues [54], but also on patients' mental well-being. Frequently, the occurrence of depression, anxiety, stress, intrusion, avoidance, and hyperarousal were observed both in patients, as well as in healthcare workers [55–59].

In the beginning of the pandemic, the Hospital of Stomatology in Wuhan diagnosed nine dental staff members infected between January to February 2020 [19]. Chinese dental surgeons responded with set of recommendations for the biosafe management of dental care workflow in the context of the epidemic [22]. Since then, various recommendations and guidelines have been published on professional websites in several countries. Most dental healthcare professionals had a high level of awareness for general COVID-19 infection prevention and control guidelines [59]. For example, guidance was provided in the US (Centers for Disease Control and Prevention (CDC), American Dental Association), in Europe (European Centre for Disease Prevention and Control (ECDC)), in France (Health Ministry, French Dental Association) and in the UK (National Health Service, British Dental Association) [60]. One of the first renowned pandemic-dental events in European dentistry was the outbreak in North Italy in Lombardy. All of Lombardy's dentists were evaluated with an online ad hoc questionnaire; 3599 questionnaires were analyzed. Of these, 502 (14.43%) participants had suffered one or more symptoms referable to COVID-19; 31 subjects were positive for the virus SARS-CoV-2 and 16 subjects developed the disease. Only a small number of dentists (n = 72, 2.00%) were confident of avoiding infection [61].

Several innovative biosafe approaches of dental diagnostics or treatment were introduced, for example telehealth solutions such as Dental Monitoring® (DM) (Dental

Monitoring Co., Paris, France) [6,62–67]. Revisions of the then-established protocols in dental healthcare were simple. Dental professionals, in their early efforts to adapt their biosafety measures, typically performed a web search conducted in the main databases of the scientific publications, focused mostly on oral rinsing and limitation of in-office aerosol production. This early research often led to possible revisions of biosafety and disinfection protocols in the dental offices [1,2]. Two years of ongoing pandemic has changed the practice of dentistry forever, and some of these changes have made dental care more time-consuming, difficult, and costly due to the possible pathways of transmission and mitigation steps needed to prevent the spread of the infection.

Despite the widespread anxiety and fear of the devastating health effects of earlier COVID-19 (2020–2021), only 61% of dentists have implemented a fundamental modification to their treatment protocols. Currently, facing the highly transmissible Omicron strains, as an urgent matter of public health, all dentists must identify the additional steps they can take to prevent the spread of air-borne infection [21].

The clinical practice biosafety guidelines, developed during the first year of the pandemic, offer recommendations which guide dental staff in providing safe dental care in the clinical environment. Such recommendations must be updated as new evidence of virus properties arises [68,69]. There is a high level of agreement between different dental specializations about the necessary preventive measures of the routes of transmission. Published data regarding the survivability of the virus on innate objects vary substantially [70]. Nevertheless, due to the wearing of personal protective equipment (respirators, gloves, masks, eye shields, and gowns) and use of disinfection procedures, this risk can be significantly mitigated. Research published by Estrich et al., found in June 2020 that during the first wave of pandemic only 0.3% of surveyed dentists had a probable COVID-19 diagnosis, of these 82.2% were asymptomatic. The most reported health problems among dentists during the pandemic were anxiety and depression [21,71].

The primary aim of most biosafety protocols is to prevent any cross-contamination while allowing the provision of urgent and emergency dental care. Aerosol-producing and other elective procedures should be avoided in the periods of outbreaks of unknown variants [17,72–75]. Various biosafety protocols detail the safety and operational measures to be taken, while providing dental care in the COVID-era. Falahchai et al. [76] published a comprehensive protocol regarding dental care during the COVID-19 outbreak. The point in the outbreaks caused by new, not well researched variants, is that these might bring dangerous long-term health hazards enabled by new mutations.

With the currently waning post-vaccination immunity worldwide, together with less cautious behavior of the general public, there is a high probability of infections providing more opportunities for further virus mutations. The Omicron variant BA.2 will only be substituted with more transmissible strain. Hopes for guaranteed declining virulence of future mutated strains are "wishful thinking" rather than an evidence-based theory. As evidence mounts that the Omicron variant is less lethal than prior strains, one of the frequently cited explanations is that viruses always evolve over time to become less virulent. This theory has already been soundly debunked. During surges of unexplored mutated variants, dental treatment might be limited to patients with urgent or emergency situations. Patients should be provided with separate waiting and operating rooms to minimize the risk of transmission of infection and treatment should be provided with the same protective measures regarding Personal Protective Equipment (PPE) for the dental clinicians and staff [76].

The last two years of pandemic in dental care showed changes in attitude from initial negligence of possible serious impacts of the virus spread, up to panic precautions. After a year, the variables of the pandemic situation have changed with the implementation of mass vaccination. This represented an important milestone [77,78], suggesting a possible end-game scenario for the COVID-19 pandemic. These expectations were facing disappointment with the arrival of the Omicron variant. The imagined race between SARS-CoV-2 mutations and vaccine rollouts was slowed down with negative perception of people afraid of possible vaccination side effects. A recent study from the Czech Republic proved the distribution of side effects among Czech healthcare workers as highly consistent with the manufacturer's data. The overall prevalence of local and systemic side effects was higher than the manufacturer's report [78]. Current data suggest that Omicron capabilities to evade natural human immunity, protective effects of distributed vaccines [79,80] and its resistance to current monoclonal medication [81,82] make the Omicron variant a true dilemma. According to a recent study by Dr Michael Chan Chi-wai, from December 2021, it can infect faster and better than Delta in human bronchus, but with a less severe infection in the lung [83]. Due to its newly gained strong ability to infect ACE2 in mice, it is predicted that this variant is here to stay until pushed out with a more transmissible strain [84].

A recent study of the American Dental Association published by Araujo et al. [23] suggests that US dentists show a high level of adherence to enhanced infection control measures in response to the ongoing pandemic, resulting in low rates of cumulative prevalence of COVID-19. With the spread of "Omicron-like" mutant strains, the likelihood of recurrent infection raises some doubts about whether vaccination alone will provide long-term immunity against COVID-19 and its future variants. Furthermore, several mutations in the receptor binding domain and S2 are predicted to impact transmissibility and affinity for ACE-2 that might be relevant for the adaptation of biosafety protocols [80].

From this perspective, the aim to provide biosafe dental workflow in orthodontic or any other dental practices must consider the higher transmissibility of the virus and higher number of asymptomatic carriers. The expectation that when the virus spreads naturally it will diminish or become less virulent is not possible, nor is it certain that further mutations will be harmless. Therefore, the effective biosafety protocol must be sustainable. Based on these facts, various simulations and modelling data, dental practices may never return to "normal", former routine operation even after global vaccination would be somehow successful as there would still be a significant risk of outbreaks of infection with new mutant strains. Variable, multi-level measures will still be required, depending on the local COVID-19 cases rate, to secure safe dental care provision [45].

Biosafety protocols, applied a year after the pandemic outbreak, are not significantly different from the ones effective today, although the virus transmissibility and symptoms have changed significantly. This work introduces a prospective setting of a combination of field-tested technologies for enhanced clinical biosafety of orthodontic workflow in confrontation with surging cases of Omicron variant infections [79,83–85]. The effectivity and sustainability of this protocol lies in its simplicity and the fact that despite new variants being more invasive to human immunity, their air-borne pathway is equally obstructed with masks, and indoor biosafety measures.

Omicron SARS-CoV-2 (B.1.1.529) and its sublineage BA.2 remain variants of concern [69,86] and they define a new chapter in the COVID-19 pandemic. This highly mutated strain has more than 30 mutations, several of which overlap with those in the Alpha, Beta, Gamma, or Delta variants of concern. These mutations and deletions are known to lead to increased transmissibility, higher viral binding affinity, and higher antibody escape. The long-term potential of the new variants is not certain yet [79–81,84,85,87–90] and preliminary research publications suggest it is from 2 to 4.2 times more infectious than the Delta variant [85]. BA.2 is more transmissible, more replicative in human nasal epithelial cells and more fusogenic than BA.1 [86]. It evades not only human natural immunity but also immunity from vaccines [84], and a number of laboratory studies have previously shown a reduced ability of approved vaccines to neutralize the new variant.

The ability of this variant to evade immunity from previous infections in contrast to the Delta and Alpha variants was presented in population-level evidence [90], and thus, this suggestion is epidemiologically important in countries with huge amounts of previously infected cases, such as Slovakia. Preliminary evidence [87,91,92] shows that there is an increased risk of reinfection of the Omicron variant and this is probably caused by Omicron escaping neutralization antibodies [93]. Even after two doses of mRNA vaccines, higher transmissibility of Omicron was also observed in Norway [94]. The booster dose may not prevent people from becoming infected, but the observed symptoms were mild or moderate [95,96]. The time since the second or booster vaccination plays a role in effectiveness against symptomatic disease, as noticed in United Kingdom [97].

Based on these evaluations of Omicron strains, each new VOC results in uncertainty; there is a struggle to reduce transmission, discuss vaccines efficacy, supply elective-care and prevent long COVID-19 complications. Thus, it is not only vaccines that play a key role in preventing COVID-19 spread, but also solutions such as biosafety protocols are complementary and highly demanded.

The risk of transmission of pathogens in the dental office resulting in an infectious disease is still unknown; it seems to be limited in developed countries, but it cannot be considered negligible [98]. Current biosafety settings are organized into five distinct areas of pandemic control, comprising:

(1) Planning and protocols;
(2) Patient screening;
(3) Preparation of facilities;
(4) PPE and infection control;
(5) Aerosol control.

Research published by Estrich et al. [71] showed that dental professionals have enhanced their infection control practices in response to COVID-19 and have benefited from a greater availability of personal protective equipment. Most practicing dentists (72.8%) used personal protective equipment according to interim guidance from the Centers for Disease Control and Prevention.

As the pandemic situation will develop towards more infectious variants, new considerations, new protocols, and new mechanisms will be implemented in the dentistry profession, including the teledentistry approach [99].

The possible lower lethality of the Omicron variant in combination with the significantly higher ability to infect and create asymptomatic carriers might be dangerous. The effects of COVID-19 are very diverse and they vary from individual to individual. Many patients develop long-term disabilities, such as pulmonary, cardiovascular, hematological, renal, gastrointestinal, reproductive, psychological, and central nervous system problems, which can last from months to years [100]. The blood–brain barrier pathway can let the virus into the neural system and cause neuronal damage as well as neurodegeneration or long-term neurological and psychosocial consequences [101–104]. Cardiovascular problems (e.g., myocarditis, arrhythmias, myocardial damage) are also quite common [105] and recent studies have shown that SARS-CoV-2 infection also affects the human reproductive system, and especially the male reproductive system via the ACE2 receptor [106,107].

This work introduces a novel combination of biosafety measures for dental workflow adaptation to preserve biosafety in dental care confronted with highly transmissible air-borne viruses. The combination of the described procedures and technologies, especially setting with UVC and virucidal air-dispersed oils, can suppress the air-borne translation of the virus and has not been investigated yet. This biosafety protocol could provide a simple and long-term sustainable model for a biosafe dental workflow, as it can manage renewed and increased risks brought by the more infectious Omicron variant carried with asymptomatic infectious patients. The present study aims to determine its clinical reliability with retrospective identification of events where a dental procedure was performed unknowingly on an infected patient, the frequency of this occurring, and cross infection incidents.

The main goal of this patient-centered study was to evaluate introduced biosafety measures for orthodontic workflow as a prospective setting for prevention of in-office infections with air-borne SARS-CoV-2 variants. The secondary goal was to provide preliminary data for a larger study.

2. Materials and Methods

2.1. Main Objective and Study Design

The study objectives were to answer whether, under this prospective setting, infected patients were treated and if any infection with SARS-CoV-2 occurred in the monitored clinical environment.

This was a single-arm, single-center small-scale study set up in a particular clinic. Data were collected after 18 months of protocol in place with a pseudonymous online form. Everyone treated in the clinic within this period experienced the same conditions.

The primary planned outcome of the study was a confirmation of exposure of the environment and personnel to infected patients with no cross infections.

Due to known limitations of single-arm studies, the conclusions of this study can be limited. On the other hand, this design was the only viable choice for investigating biosafety measures, as the non-application of any preventive measures in pandemic would not be ethical. Alternatives for external control groups for this single-arm trial were considered; however, there is no comparative data available about how frequently patients become infected during orthodontic appointments.

2.2. Participants and the Environment

The protocol was applied and evaluated in the clinical environment of dental clinic with 4 doctors, 4 dental nurses and one manager.

During an 18-month evaluation period, approximately 2500 appointments were scheduled in a digital calendar for 160 different patients, not including their accompanying persons. Approximately 2230 appointments took place (others were cancelled or postponed mostly due to pandemic health precautions or travel complications).

The environment for dental care consists of fully separable rooms with independent air processing and separate Ultraviolet—C light (UVC) air sterilization systems. Each of the three rooms have an independent dental unit with a separate nurse position.

2.3. Brief Description of the Protocol

The key attributes of this biosafety protocol are:

- Efficient;
- Sustainable;
- Simple;
- Applicable in other dental specialties (despite orthodontic customization).

The fundamental backbone of this protocol is a combination of air treatment and new technologies. Air treatment is performed with a combination of hooded UVC sterilization and air disinfection with the creation of a virucidal air puffer made by a certified virucidal oil nebulizer/diffuser. Key technologies implemented as part of this protocol in the workflow are artificial intelligence in patient diagnostics, continuous and post-treatment monitoring, smart mobile patient coaching, 3D printing for aerosol control and some other techs.

The set-up of this protocol might be considered as a biosafety overkill; however, the current risks of airborne infection that could come from an asymptomatic carrier and circumvent immune defenses, causing a permanent health damage to someone else, is not negligible. With future, more transmissible, variants to come, professional dedication to preserving the highest biosafety level in the dental office and efficient air processing protocols will be needed.

This protocol is intended as a possible complement to existing methodologies. It represents more than a year of our interdisciplinary efforts dedicated to clinical testing and the implementation of various new technologies and working procedures to maintain the biosafety of dental healthcare. Dental care must be provided taking into consideration the patient safety as well as the safety of healthcare professionals.

This protocol was created as part of an interdisciplinary cooperation of epidemiologists, infectologists, dental surgeons, general dentists, orthodontists, and other healthcare professionals. It provides inspiration for wider clinical implementation and assessment. It is our contribution to solving this historical situation affecting safety and availability of oral care.

The fundamental principle of this protocol is full room volume air treatment with a combination of UVC and virucidal oil diffusion. Sterilization of the entire volume of air (for each patient) of the given treatment unit (room) by a combination of a UVC light and a created permanent virucidal buffer of certified disinfectant oils and special active FFP3 protective aids. The key additions to the protocol are fundamental changes in working practices in the provision of artificial intelligence and telemedicine. There are two main parts of the permanent daily protocol:

- Full room-volume air UVC sterilization for each patient * total air volume per dental unit (separated room);
- Permanent air dispersed super small droplets of virucide oil—a protective puffer in recommended concentrations, created with disinfectant fogging machine (nebulizer).

Complementary technologies for digital workflow:

- AI video-scan evaluation (common checkups rendered obsolete)—Dental Monitoring;
- custom made IOS/Android app coaching the proper habits—StrojCHECK [12];
- 3D printed aerosol vacuum pump ending, that supports aerosol dispersion during dental procedures and other customized 3D printing allowing more.

2.4. *Comprehensive Biosafety Protocol Description*

2.4.1. Introduction and the Focus of the Protocol

The aim of this protocol was to define safe and, at the same time, physically and economically sustainable measures for a longer period of the pandemic with the minimization of the impact on the provided healthcare in dental practice. The objective was to maintain a high quality of care, without a significant increase in the costs and with no tolerance to any exposure of the staff or patients.

Work on this protocol began on 6 February 2020, and it took us more than 9 months to experiment, test, and implement various new practices, technologies, and modifications to existing practices. Through final consultations with experts, it has taken on its present form. This protocol can be currently considered as useful and inspiring for clinicians looking for cost-effective solutions that can be sustainable in the long run. Despite all our staff being vaccinated, with the Omicron variant, they might be infectious and simultaneously not show clinical symptoms [79–83,85,87–90].

New and improved procedures have been implemented to develop this protocol in cooperation with renowned infectologists, epidemiologists and other experts. Examples of some implemented technological innovations are:

1. Online dynamic anamnestic forms (effectively replacing part of 4D clinical examinations);
2. Teledentistry Teleorthodontics—Dental Monitoring® (DM) (Dental Monitoring Co., Paris, France)/https://dental-monitoring.com/ (accessed on 1 December 2021) and (StrojCHECK®, Bratislava, Slovakia, 3Dent Medical, www.osim.sk (accessed on 1 December 2021) [12];
3. Artificial intelligence in telediagnostics—active screening of patients in tandem with the doctor;
4. Special medical devices—active FFP3 shield respirator, BioVYZR, Toronto USA-based Vyzr Technologies, a shield that covers the wearer's face and protects against droplets and pathogens. Powered Air Purifying Respirator (PAPR), a device typically used only in industrial and healthcare settings;
5. 3D printing of sterilizable devices (aerosol aspirators for surgical aspirators or individualized handles);
6. Two-phase air sterilization (diffusers of biocidal oils with UVC, NewAroma.sk).

2.4.2. The Protocol Principles

This protocol does not inevitably change the procedures already established so far for sterilization of dental instruments, disinfection of surfaces and other routinely applied rules of each dental clinic. These remain, as the current pandemic is just one of the many infections we fight in asepsis in the dental clinic environment. Its key set of differences from HIV, EBV, HSV and other common viruses is the period of possible asymptomatic air-borne transmissibility. The advantage of modern orthodontic therapy with clear aligners is the relatively rare occurrence of the need for urgent treatment. In the case of urgent orthodontic treatment of a confirmed infectious COVID-19 patient, a bio-hazard protocol is applied as in HIV patients, in COVID-19 with an emphasis on the prevention of airborne spread. Regardless of whether the treatment involves aerosol dispersion (e.g., removal of attachments or fixed retainer or orthodontic auxiliaries such as distalizer, power-arms [108,109] or power caps), the treatment procedure differs from the standard protocol only in the fact that the patient has the last appointment of the day shift—as the last procedure on a given day.

Oral rinsing is not routinely recommended in our protocol for all patients. Only in the patients where intra-oral procedure is planned, iodine prerinse for 30 s is indicated. Rinsing does not address the nasopharyngeal region with the largest "virus load" (reported in the nasopharynx). From our practical experience, the recommended 30 s rinsing often led to a "run-in" and subsequent coughing of the patient and thus unnecessary contamination of the space. This protocol recommends careful rinsing only while attachments are being replaced or cleaned, during bio3dir removal and "powerCaps", "powerArms" removal, interproximal recontouring or dental hygiene procedures. Prior to these procedures, the patient rinses the mouth for 30 s.

This protocol works on the premise that either patient, nurse or doctor are infectious. This is the reason the protocol includes:

1. Minimization of time exposure (shortened duration of treatment, replacement of unnecessary physical visits of the patient via AV technologies, ordering for the exact time with preparation of everything necessary for the procedure in advance).
2. Mechanical and physic-chemical prevention in the dispersion of the virus and its carriers into the space resp. decontamination (PPE, continuous sterilization of the air and virucide "puffer" in the air) et al.
3. Preventive (patient input filter—symptoms, smart-App tracking, continuous testing of healthcare professionals).

A slightly elevated temperature that is acceptable under this protocol is 37.8 °C (originally taken from CDC). The uniforms of the medical staff are rotated daily. They include all surface clothing including shoes and socks. No hazmat suits are used.

2.4.3. Brief Description of Technologies Utilized in the Protocol

The protocol implements the following technologies and practices:

1. Online dynamic anamnestic forms;
2. Artificial intelligence in dental monitoring;
3. Robotization of automatic surface disinfection;
4. A.I. smart patient app for treatment coaching;
5. 3D printing of sterilizable devices;
6. Regular COVID-19 testing of personnel;
7. UVC and diffused virucidal oil air treatment.

1. The use of online dynamic anamnestic smart forms such as Typeform (www.typeform.com, accessed on 18 May 2022) brings interactivity and order to communication with patients at home. The idea of online dynamic anamnestic forms is to use the patient's own mobile phone not only for video communication (WhatsApp, Facetime), but also for outsourcing part of the examination. For example, with the proper instructions, a short selfie/video sequence of a natural smile can be captured by the patient and

provided within an online smart form. The anamnesis itself is very important in reducing the risk of transmission, the proportion of asymptomatic patients with COVID-19 was less than 30% in the number of children with the highest proportion of asymptomatic infection. The identification of symptomatic patients is the first and relatively most effective method of risk reduction. Since the anamnesis is taken remotely, neither staff nor co-patients are exposed to the risk of infection, nor is there any contamination of the surfaces in the waiting room. The use of dynamic forms from Typeform is a suitable choice for this protocol. Remote screening of COVID-19 symptoms by application has been identified as a suitable method for detecting COVID-19 infection. Even the survey form for this biosafety protocol clinical evaluation was created as a smart form. It asks a set of questions that differs according to the answers given. The logic behind it is shown in Figure 1.

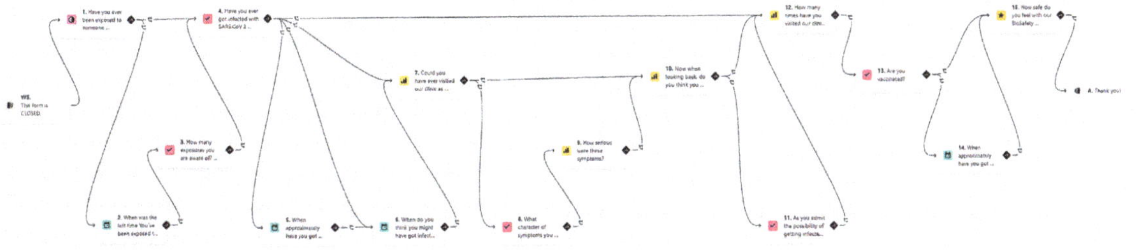

Figure 1. Example of logic behind the online smart form. English version of the survey evaluation in this protocol. URL: https://sangreazul.typeform.com/BioSafety-ENG (accessed on 15 December 2021).

2. Artificial intelligence (AI) technology implemented in the form of the Dental Monitoring software uses the patient's mobile phone for regular "scanning", either to assess the course of treatment or to screen a growing patient by monitoring their development or monitoring retention stability after cessation of treatment. A special holder allows the patient to record a video of their own teeth. Paradoxically, it allows more regular and even more thorough inspection, as using artificial intelligence allowed us to summon the patient to an appointment only when necessary (Figure 2). Each video scan first evaluates using AI and then it alerts the doctor only to the monitored situations. The form of our workflow has thus changed fundamentally, and healthcare professionals spend a large part of the day reviewing the outputs of artificial intelligence, which, in turn, extremely efficiently evaluates huge volumes of data, such as video scans of our patients' oral cavities. It is not humanly possible to evaluate the hundreds of video scans that patients regularly make. The "brute force" of this technology is ideal for identifying situations requiring human intervention.
3. Robotized around-the-clock surface disinfection technology is also used. It should respect all existing guidelines with an emphasis on consistency and differentiation of surfaces and a higher frequency of cleaning (after each patient). After entering, the patient should only be in contact with the necessary surfaces, and disinfect her/his hands first. Frequent cleaning of surfaces in the clinic, after each procedure, should include frequently inspected surfaces such as door handles, keyboards, and mice. There is also the addition of floor cleaning by robotic vacuuming with a disinfection mop, in our case, the iRobot Braava jet m6, which is suitable for up to 100 m^2. The CDC recommends applying standard virucidal disinfectants to potentially contaminated surfaces to prevent the spread of SARS-CoV-2 infection. The work on the susceptibility of human coronaviruses and SARS-CoV is expected to be highly effective in SARS-CoV-2, which is relatively resistant to environmental conditions and remains infectious on smooth surfaces such as metal and plastic for many days.

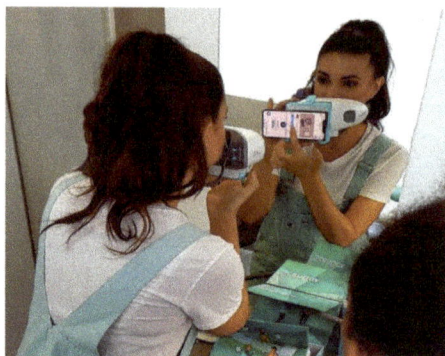

Figure 2. First Dental Monitoring session, in which the patient is educated with the nurse about how to use the free app in his/her own mobile in combination with the "scanbox" holder. Published with written consent of the person.

4. Self-developed smart mobile application technology is used for patient treatment coaching and remote discipline support. The authors of this paper have been gradually developing iterations of the free telehealth smart patient application for patients in orthodontic treatment with clear aligners, to support proper habits/stereotypes. This app allows for better remote management of the patient and possible reduction in the frequency of visits to the dental office. The application educates and motivates the patient to behave responsibly [12]. For example, the app provides motivation and coaching for more frequent cleaning of teeth and aligners and in general it improved patient compliance.
5. 3D printing technology supports the presented biosafety protocol with specific sterilizable aerosol aspirators (Figure 3A–D). These devices are printed by a MultiJet Fusion 3D Pro Printer and are sterilizable at 121 °C in autoclave. This aerosol interception device is called "SUR-FACE" and was developed by an Italian orthodontist because of the COVID-19 pandemic. It connects to a conventional 16 mm suction device. The material is polyamide and is compatible with any retractor with thickness ≤ 2 mm. The material is recyclable and supplied with five additional rubber seals. The one-time use of suction cup attachments minimizes the risk of transmitting infection with this tool. The sterilizability of these handpieces is critical. From clinical experience, it is very effective at containing aerosols produced during clinical procedures.
6. Regular antigen testing from saliva or other convenient form of testing for possible infectiousness of everybody in the team shall be employed because, with the arrival of Omicron-like strains, it is even more likely that a vaccinated healthcare professional would become a "supercarrier".
7. Air-processing technologies are key to the presented biosafety protocol with two-phase air treatment: room air is the most likely vector and therefore a key element in the stopping of transmission of infection. The transmission of SARS-CoV-2 infection occurs mainly through droplets that fall relatively rapidly to the ground. However, aerosolized particles smaller than 5 µm contaminate the air and can levitate indoors where the air is not exchanged and disinfected for several hours. In addition to PPE, aerosol extractors and other elements preventing significant air contamination in the clinic, it is therefore appropriate to include other forms of air conditioning, in our case hooded UVC emitters combined with diffusers of biocidal oils, suitable for combination with UVC sterilization.

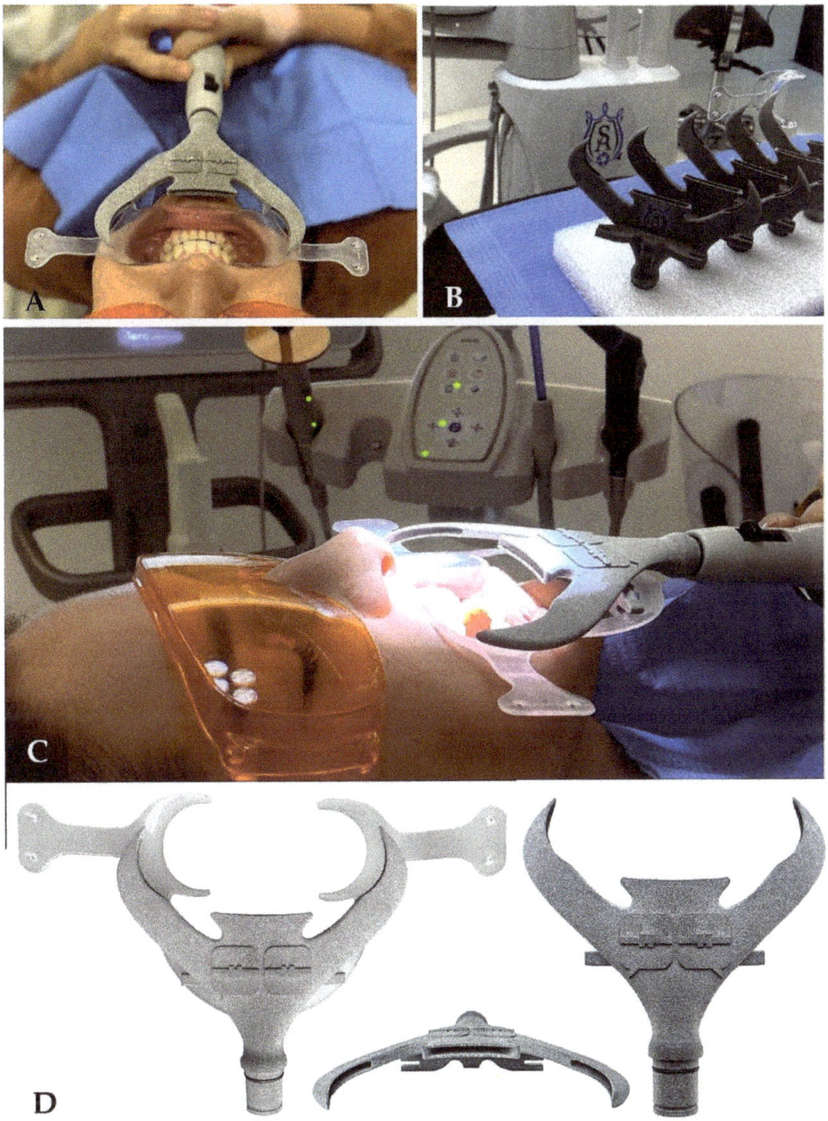

Figure 3. 3D printed aerosol interception device. (**A**) Frontal view of 3D printed aerosol suction attached to surgical suction system and oral retractor. (**B**) With 3D printing, each office can be supported with adequate quantities. (**C**) Lateral view of "SUR-FACE" attached to conventional retractor. (**D**) View of "SUR-FACE" with and without cheek retractor and view of three suction openings.

2.4.4. Air-Processing Elements (UVC + Virucidal Diffusers)

Sterilization of the entire air volume of one separate room in clinic with volume of 13 m^3 will take approximately 25~30 min (time intervals between patients). SARS-CoV-2 virus particles are rapidly inactivated by UVC radiation. Two hardware key elements of the presented prospective biosafety setting are UVC and Diffuser.

(A) Germicidal radiator PROLUX G30W A/SPH01:

- UVC lamp life of 8000 h;

- For two-shift operation endurance 550 days (2 × 7.5 h);
- 1 emitter cycle is sufficient to sterilize a volume of 5.5 m × 4 m × 3.0 m;

(B) Aroma Pro Mini—professional diffuser (aroma atomizer).

- For air conditioning;
- Capacity up to 1000 m^3 (www.NewAroma.sk accessed on 15 December 2021);
- Possibility to choose from several certified disinfectant oils;
- Disinfectant is present in the mixture in 3 weight percent at an emission of 5 mL per hour (adjustable) to form an invisible aerosol dispersion in the air.

2.5. Protocol Development and Evaluation

The protocol has been in development from 8 February 2020 until 1 June 2020 (5 months). The unchanged protocol in place was from 1 June 2020 until 30 November (18 months). The protocol evaluation with auto-locked online smart forms was performed between 1 December and 12 December.

2.6. Protocol strengths and Weaknesses

Strengths:

- Low cost, affordable, effective, sustainable
- Does not require specific rebuilding of the current dental set-ups
- Dimensioned for highly transmissible strains coming after Omicron
- Not dependable on vaccination status or unreliable testing results

Weaknesses:

- Difficult to evaluate clinical reliability:
  - The only possible way is feedback form (bias);
  - Larger sample needed;
  - Other studies for comparison are needed;
- Requiring extra time gaps between patients in the same room;
- Possible biosafety overkill;
- Unknown performance under unexplored highly transmissible variants.

3. Results

3.1. Descriptive Results

From 160 relevant patients, the online smart form was filled out and submitted 115 times. There were eight responses in English the rest were in Slovak. The special fingerprint feature identified three duplicate answers that were removed. The result was 111 valid responses (69.37%). All answers are in the table that is available online in the public repository.

Approximately half of the responding patients were exposed to an infected person with COVID-19 (Figure 4). From 111 patients, exactly 56 (50 5%) were directly exposed to SARS-Co-2 infection and 55 (49 5%) were not (during the last 18 months). Dates of these exposures are shown in Figure 5.

Of the responding patients, 90 (81%) were vaccinated (Figure 6 and Table 1); however, only 14 had had a Pfizer booster (3rd) shot.

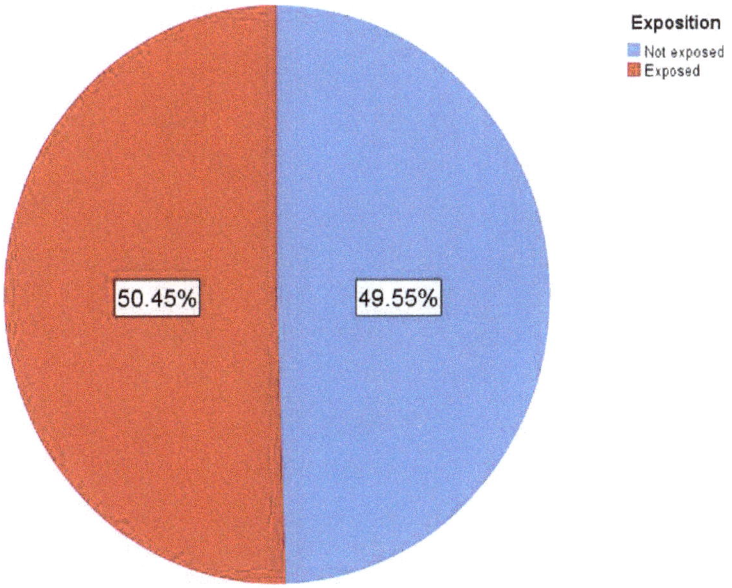

Figure 4. This graph represents distribution of exposed vs. non exposed patients to someone diagnosed with COVID-19 during the last 18 months.

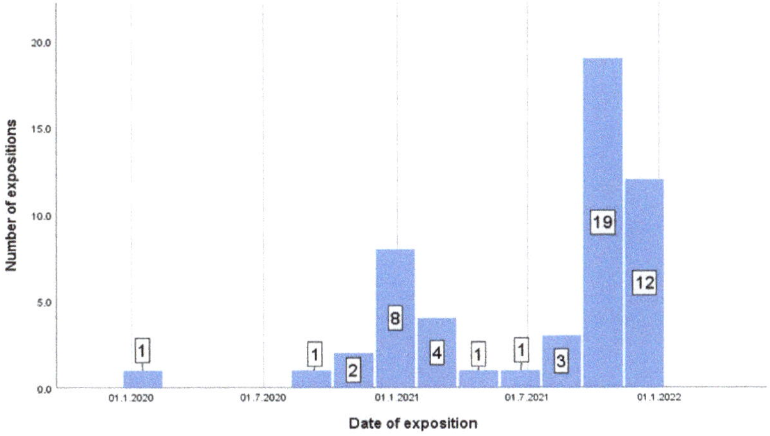

Figure 5. Frequency of exposure to an infected person by the date.

Table 1. Vaccination status of all responses.

Status	Frequency	Percent
not vaccinated	21	18.9
vaccinated	90	81.1
Total	111	100.0

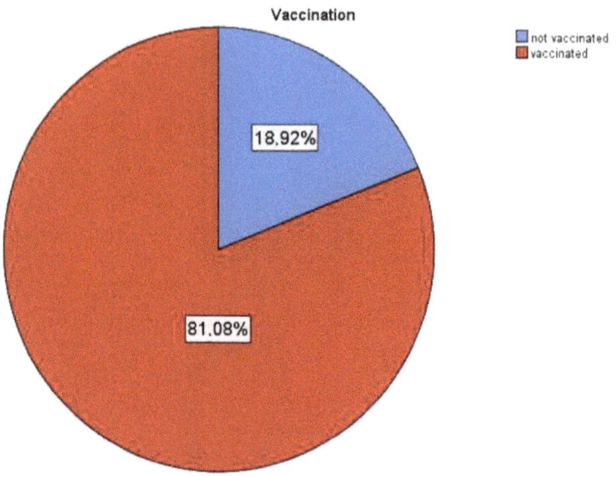

Figure 6. Vaccination distribution in patients.

Fifty-eight were vaccinated with two shots of Pfizer, seven with Moderna, four with Janssen and eight with AstraZeneca.

Forty-five (50%) of all vaccinated patients received their last shot until June 2021.

Nine patients reported the possibility of being infectious during their visit at the clinic.

Thirty-eight responders got infected with the SARS-CoV.2 virus.

Thirty- seven responders rejected the possibility that they got infected at the clinic under the evaluated protocol. Only one of them considered this as the possibility with the lowest offered level of confidence.

Regarding the question about the feeling of biosafety experienced by the patients during the dental procedure (Figure 7), the patients' feelings were evaluated on a scale from 1 to 5, where the 1 represents "no safety feeling" to 5 "very safe". From 111 patients, the mean feeling was M = 4.59, SD = 0.732.

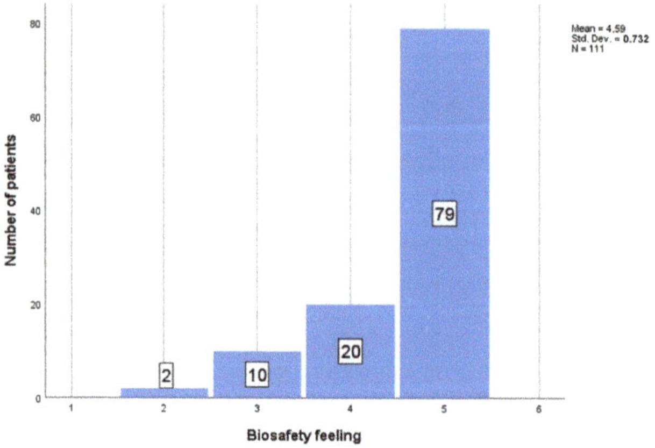

Figure 7. Biosafety feeling records by value.

Thirty-seven patients answered the question "Could you have ever visited our clinic already infected?" (Figure 8). The scale available was from 1 (*no, there was no chance of being infectious during the visit*) to 5 (*yes, I was infectious during the visit*). M = 1.32, SD = 0.818. All the infectious patients visiting the clinic were asymptomatic, as otherwise they would not have got through the initial entry filter (Figure 9).

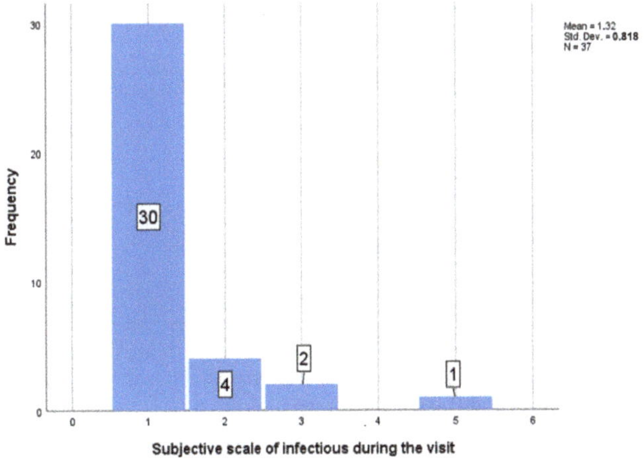

Figure 8. Number of subjective infectious status during visit.

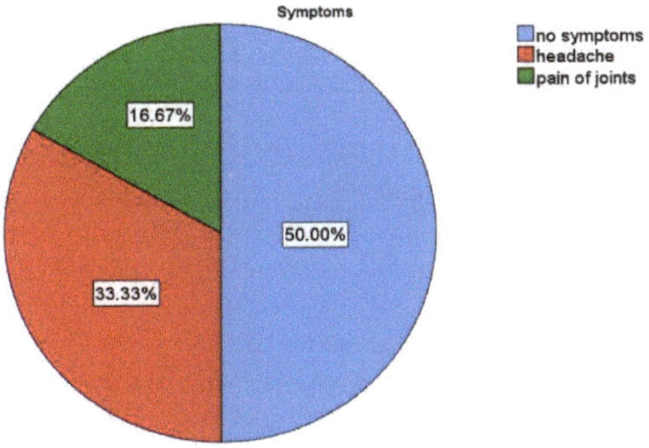

Figure 9. Potential infectious patients during the visit and spectrum of their symptoms.

3.2. Graphical Interpretation of Clinical Evaluation of the Protocol

Out of 111 patients, 56 (50.5%) were exposed to SARS-Co-2 infection and 55 (49.5%) were not (Figure 4). The incidence of exposure to an infected person is shown in Figure 5.

The one-sample t test revealed a significant difference in the distribution of the exposures t (51) = 7,103,185, $p < 0.001$ during the time (M = 14.7.2021; SD = 162 d).

The independent sample t test showed the significantly higher number of exposures in the unvaccinated group (N = 11, M = 3.91, SD = 1.3) compared to in the vaccinated group (N = 45; M = 2.42, SD = 1.438) t (54) = 3.127, p = 0.003.

There was no significant correlation and a low Pearson's correlation (almost significant) between the date of exposition and number of the protentional contacts with SARS-Co-2 r = 0.265, N = 52, p = 0.058.

3.3. Biosafety Protocol

The safety feeling of the patients was recorded on a scale from 1 to 5, where the 1 represents "no safety feeling" to 5 "very safe"; from 111 patients, the mean feeling was M = 4.59, SD = 0.732 (see Figure 7 and Table 2).

Between the two groups of unvaccinated patients—one of which was named "Never got the vaccine against SARS-Co-2" (N = 5, M = 5, SD = 0) and the other was "Unvaccinated, but still waiting" (N = 16, M = 4.5, SD = 0.730)—there was no significant difference between the biosafety feeling t (19) = −1.504, p = 0.149.

Table 2. Biosafety feeling of patients during dental procedures, full data available in supplementary materials.

	N	Mean	Std. Deviation	Std. Error	95% Confidence Interval for Mean Lower Bound	95% Confidence Interval for Mean Upper Bound	Minimum	Maximum
disease free	74	4.55	0.743	0.086	4.38	4.73	2	5
Ab +	3	4.67	0.577	0.333	3.23	6.10	4	5
PCR/Ag +	30	4.73	0.583	0.106	4.52	4.95	3	5
multiple	3	3.67	1.528	0.882	−0.13	7.46	2	5
other	1	5.00	0.0	0.0	0.0	0.0	5	5
Total	111	4.59	0.732	0.069	4.45	4.72	2	5

There was no statistical difference in biosafety feeling between the group of vaccinated patients and the patients who had not had a booster dose (N = 78, M = 4.56, SD = 0.783) and those who had had a booster dose (N = 12, M = 4.67, SD = 0.492).

Thirty-seven patients answered the question "Could you have ever visited our clinic as already infected?". There was scale, which divided the risk of infectious status to 1 (no, there were no chance to be infectious during the visit), to 5 (yes, I was infectious during the visit) M = 1.32, SD = 0.818.

Of the patients who answered the question of possible infectious status during the visit (N = 6) (scale of potential risk was higher than 1), most recorded that they had no symptoms during the visit N = 3 (50%), but others noted that they had headache N = 2 (33.3%) and pain of joints N = 1 (16.67%) (Figures 8 and 9).

There was medium correlation between number of exposures and potentially infectious patients r (28) = 0.402; $p = 0.034$.

4. Discussion

The evaluated prospective setting for orthodontic workflow is based on a combination of well-researched technologies and known virucidal effects. Together, this combination is simple and sustainable. Despite the results, which preliminarily suggest its virucidal effectivity of such a prospective setting, these shall be considered as preliminary data for a larger study.

Evaluated subjective feedback from pseudonymous questionnaires showed that, under this prospective setting, infected patients were treated with high probability. Additionally, data suggest that chances of SARS-CoV-2 cross infection occurrence in the monitored clinical environment were extremely low.

With an awareness of the limitations of single-arm, single-center studies, it shall be emphasized that practice guidelines should rarely, if ever, be based on evidence from single-center trials and this study shall encourage clinicians from the dental community to engage in further and wider evaluation of such prospective settings. The combination of UVC and dispersed oil in virucidal air-processing might evolve in the very near future to a sustainable model for biosafe dental care. Dispersion of aerosols during dental therapy and other procedures and technologies to reduce the contagion among dentists have been well researched [7,110,111]. However, there is currently no comparative data available about how frequently patients become infected during orthodontic appointments or other biosafety efficiency.

Further interpretation of the study results shows that from 115 online form responses, one was probably intentionally invalid as it repeatedly referred to triple vaccination even before third shots were available in the EU, as well as references to events out of the observed 18-month period and it entered various other oxymorons. This response has been evaluated as invalid.

Approximately every second responder had a history of recent COVID-19 exposition. Dates of these exposures (Figure 5) correlate with the Slovak regional pandemic situation and it is clear to see the difference between the previous and the current wave.

Forty-five (50%) of all vaccinated responders received their last shot before June 2021, so with over 6 months since last vaccination, their immunity from vaccines against the Omicron variant will not be probably relevant.

The evaluation of the protocol reveals nine patients reporting the possibility of them being infectious during their visit to the clinic. There was no incident of personnel becoming infected by patients or within work. Only two of the personnel were infected with COVID-19 in the past. Both cases were from well-known family sources.

Of the 38 infected responders, 37 rejected the possibility that they were infected at the clinic in the monitored period. Only one of them considered this as a possibility, but with the lowest offered level of confidence. There were five levels of confidence in this parameter:

1. Certainly not! 0%;
2. 25%;
3. Maybe, 50%;
4. 75%;
5. I am sure I got it there 100%.

Thirty-seven patients answered the question "Could you have ever visited our clinic already infected?" (Figure 8). All the infectious patients visiting the clinic were asymptomatic, as they would not have got through the initial entry filter (Figure 9).

In this paper, the authors have presented a biosafety protocol with further context to orthodontic care facing the Omicron variant with new epidemiological properties. With this new variant, a higher transmissibility and lower protection from vaccines can be anticipated, albeit with possibly milder clinical symptoms [79,81–85,87,89,90]. So, there will be more likelihood of having an asymptomatic carrier in a dental procedure in the near future than there is today.

The results of the survey have demonstrated that patient entry-symptomatic-screening prevented symptomatic patients present in the dental procedures. Survey also revealed that most of the vaccinated patients have probably very low or nearly no protection from vaccines [45,77,79,81,112].

The weakness of this study is the clinical evaluation of the clinical performance of the true safety of this biosafety protocol. The online survey does not show a representative sample; it depends on the self-assessment of the responders. Additionally, there is a high probability that responders are the more responsible part of the targeted group.

The results can be interpreted from the perspective of previous studies presented in the Introduction chapter as supporting the validity of the protocol. While they do not prove it to be safe, they do prove that it is not unsafe. Wider and multicentric research is necessary to prove the reliability of these settings. Ideally, research should be carried out with similar clinics not following the protocol, but working in the similar geographical location and intensity.

Approximately half of the responding patients were exposed to person infected with COVID-19; however, this is self-assessment evaluation. It is interesting that the dates of these exposures correlate with the Slovak regional pandemic situation in those times. It is also an obvious difference between the previous and the current wave. The frequency of exposures during the current wave is higher than in the previous one, when more strict lockdowns were implied. Fifty percent of all vaccinated patients had received their last shot before June 2021, so with over 6 months since the last vaccination, their immunity from vaccines against the Omicron variant will not be probably relevant [45,81].

The more transmissible Omicron variant defines a new chapter of the COVID-19 pandemic. As it is spreading at a rate unseen with any of the previous variants, there is a concern that people are dismissing Omicron as mild, not learning from the recent past. Even if Omicron does cause less severe disease, the sheer number of cases could once again overwhelm unprepared health systems [113].

Omicron contains mutations associated with higher levels of immune escape, higher transmissibility, and an improved ability to bind cells. However, there are also many mutations within the new variant that are not yet understood. As the experts have no idea what these new mutations do yet, it is logical to stay cautious and responsible [113].

Predictions of the practicality and efficiency of this prospective setting for dental care are difficult, as they face only the preliminary findings about the Omicron variant, and society's attitudes are changing. Experts are currently facing considerations of Omicron as a possible pandemic-ender, with some people including some politicians willing to take the risk for the sake of the economy. Some people are even willing to voluntarily be infected, despite the Omicron variant's known risks of infection, such as impact on the nervous system, heart tissue or the risk of long COVID-19 are known. It remains unclear whether Omicron will have any of the "silent" effects seen with earlier variants, such as self-attacking antibodies, sperm impairments and changes in insulin-producing cells.

Only time will reveal if there are other hidden risks for our health. In this regard, only recently have researchers found strong evidence that it is an infection with the Epstein–Barr virus—a particularly ubiquitous member of the herpesvirus family, best known for causing mononucleosis and triggering multiple sclerosis (MS). Infection with Epstein–Barr increased the likelihood of developing multiple sclerosis, by more than 32-fold [114].

However, as this new era puts current vaccines into a different perspective, masks, ventilation, and hygiene remain unaffected. Vaccines are tools that have the greatest impact when they are used to protect those who are most at risk. They are the last line of our defense. Today, vaccines cannot be considered as a substitute for masks, distancing, ventilation, or hand hygiene. It also seems logical that Omicron-like strains are here to stay. It can be fought with measures that work today and that must be sustainable. This presented biosafety protocol addresses higher risks suggested by preliminary observations that indicate that Omicron spreads faster and escapes antibodies more readily than previous variants. Loss of smell and taste is clinically frequent in older variants; now, with Omicron, sore throat and night sweats are reported frequently. The protocol anticipates that an increase in reinfections and cases of mild breakthrough infections in people who are vaccinated is highly probable [89].

5. Conclusions

A clinical evaluation of the introduced prospective biosafety settings for dental care and education suggests a possible sustainable solution for the next pandemic season.

The results of this work indicate the perspective application of combined procedures and technologies focused particularly on virucidal air-processing with UVC and oil dispersion as well as other technologies such as AI and telemedicine in confrontation with air-borne SARS-CoV-2 variants.

The presented prospective setting in prevention of COVID-19 was evaluated using 111 responses, suggesting that nine patients were treated as infectious asymptomatic carriers (with high probability), but no cross infection has been identified.

Despite the results suggesting the virucidal effectivity of this sustainable biosafety prospective setting, these shall be considered only as preliminary data for a larger study. Recognizing the limitations of single-arm, single-center studies, it shall be highlighted that practice guidelines should rarely, if ever, be based on evidence from single-center trials and this study shall encourage clinicians from the dental community to engage in further and wider evaluation of described technologies and procedures.

While more infectious Omicron-like strains do appear to be clinically less severe compared to Delta, their long-term effects are still unknown and dental professionals must not risk patients' infection [115].

Supplementary Materials: The following are available online at https://docs.google.com/spreadsheets/d/1lznYWB32gTb282v4HJbQRY_Uw42xXnBhNj-vnmvJvKE/edit?usp=sharing (accessed on 18 May 2022).

Author Contributions: Conceptualization, M.M. and B.N.; Data curation, A.T. and B.G.; Formal analysis, A.T., I.W., V.K., B.G. and B.N.; Funding acquisition, H.K.; Investigation, I.W.; Methodology, A.T., I.W., V.K., B.M., B.G. and M.M.; Project administration, I.V. and B.N.; Resources, A.T., W.U.; Software, A.T., I.W. and B.M.; Supervision, I.W. and B.N.; Validation, H.K. and B.G.; Visualization, A.T., I.W., B.M. and B.G.; Writing—original draft, A.T., I.V., W.U., H.K., B.M. and B.G.; Writing—review and editing, A.T., I.W., W.U., V.K., H.K. and B.M. All authors have read and agreed to the published version of the manuscript.

Funding: Data analysis was supported by The Slovak Research and Development Agency (APVV): SK-BY-RD-19-0019 and The Cultural and Educational Grant Agency of the Ministry of Education, Science, Research, and Sport of the Slovak Republic (KEGA): 041UK-4/2020.

Institutional Review Board Statement: The study was conducted according to the guidelines of the Declaration of Helsinki, and no approval was necessary by the Ethics Committee. Ethical review and approval were waived for this study since no experimental materials or approaches were used. All used materials and machines were fully certified and are still available on the market.

Informed Consent Statement: Written informed consent was obtained from all subjects involved in the study.

Data Availability Statement: We fully adhere to Data Availability Statements in section "MDPI Research Data Policies".

Acknowledgments: We acknowledge the support from experts in the fields of epidemiology, infectiology, health analytics and dentistry. Namely: Alexandra Bražinová, Neda Markovská Peter Sabaka, Ladislav Czakó, Martin Smatana, Jana Kaiferová, Martin Strunga and Renáta Urban. We acknowledge technological support of the digital Dental lab infrastructure of 3Dent Medical s.r.o company as well as dental clinic Sangre Azul s.r.o.

Conflicts of Interest: The authors declare no conflict of interest.

References

1. Siles-Garcia, A.A.; Alzamora-Cepeda, A.G.; Atoche-Socola, K.J.; Peña-Soto, C.; Arriola-Guillén, L.E. Biosafety for Dental Patients During Dentistry Care After COVID-19: A Review of the Literature. *Disaster Med. Public Health Prep.* **2021**, *15*, e43–e48. [CrossRef] [PubMed]
2. Cabrera-Tasayco, F.D.P.; Rivera-Carhuavilca, J.M.; Atoche-Socola, K.J.; Peña-Soto, C.; Arriola-Guillén, L.E. Biosafety Measures at the Dental Office After the Appearance of COVID-19: A Systematic Review. *Disaster Med. Public Health Prep.* **2020**, *15*, e34–e38. [CrossRef] [PubMed]
3. Hocková, B.; Riad, A.; Valky, J.; Šulajová, Z.; Stebel, A.; Slávik, R.; Bečková, Z.; Pokorná, A.; Klugarová, J.; Klugar, M. Oral Complications of ICU Patients with COVID-19: Case-Series and Review of Two Hundred Ten Cases. *J. Clin. Med.* **2021**, *10*, 581. [CrossRef] [PubMed]
4. Huth, K.C.; von Bronk, L.; Kollmuss, M.; Lindner, S.; Durner, J.; Hickel, R.; Draenert, M.E. Special Teaching Formats during the COVID-19 Pandemic—A Survey with Implications for a Crisis-Proof Education. *J. Clin. Med.* **2021**, *10*, 5099. [CrossRef] [PubMed]
5. Feher, B.; Wieser, C.; Lukes, T.; Ulm, C.; Gruber, R.; Kuchler, U. The Effect of the COVID-19 Pandemic on Patient Selection, Surgical Procedures, and Postoperative Complications in a Specialized Dental Implant Clinic. *J. Clin. Med.* **2022**, *11*, 855. [CrossRef]
6. Sycinska-Dziarnowska, M.; Maglitto, M.; Woźniak, K.; Spagnuolo, G. Oral Health and Teledentistry Interest during the COVID-19 Pandemic. *J. Clin. Med.* **2021**, *10*, 3532. [CrossRef]
7. Sinjari, B.; Rexhepi, I.; Santilli, M.; D'addazio, G.; Chiacchiaretta, P.; Di Carlo, P.; Caputi, S. The Impact of COVID-19 Related Lockdown on Dental Practice in Central Italy—Outcomes of A Survey. *Int. J. Environ. Res. Public Health* **2020**, *17*, 5780. [CrossRef]
8. Goriuc, A.; Sandu, D.; Tatarciuc, M.; Luchian, I. The Impact of the COVID-19 Pandemic on Dentistry and Dental Education: A Narrative Review. *Int. J. Environ. Res. Public Health* **2022**, *19*, 2537. [CrossRef]
9. Cummins, C.P.; Ajayi, O.J.; Mehendale, F.V.; Gabl, R.; Viola, I.M. The dispersion of spherical droplets in source–sink flows and their relevance to the COVID-19 pandemic. *Phys. Fluids* **2020**, *32*, 083302. [CrossRef]
10. Javaid, M.; Haleem, A.; Singh, R.P.; Suman, R. Dentistry 4.0 technologies applications for dentistry during COVID-19 pandemic. *Sustain. Oper. Comput.* **2021**, *2*, 87–96. [CrossRef]
11. Pai, S.; Patil, V.; Kamath, R.; Mahendra, M.; Singhal, D.K.; Bhat, V. Work-life balance amongst dental professionals during the COVID-19 pandemic—A structural equation modelling approach. *PLoS ONE* **2021**, *16*, e0256663. [CrossRef] [PubMed]
12. Thurzo, A.; Kurilová, V.; Varga, I. Artificial Intelligence in Orthodontic Smart Application for Treatment Coaching and Its Impact on Clinical Performance of Patients Monitored with AI-TeleHealth System. *Healthcare* **2021**, *9*, 1695. [CrossRef] [PubMed]
13. Abdelrahim, R.K.; Abdoun, H.A.E.; Koppolu, P.; Swapna, L.A. Infection Control Measures in Dental Clinics during Coronavirus Disease-19 Pandemic in Kingdom of Saudi Arabia: A Pilot Study. *Open Access Maced. J. Med Sci.* **2021**, *9*, 61–67. [CrossRef]

14. Campus, G.; Diaz-Betancourt, M.; Cagetti, M.; Carvalho, J.; Carvalho, T.; Cortés-Martinicorena, J.; Deschner, J.; Douglas, G.; Giacaman, R.; Machiulskiene, V.; et al. Study Protocol for an Online Questionnaire Survey on Symptoms/Signs, Protective Measures, Level of Awareness and Perception Regarding COVID-19 Outbreak among Dentists. A Global Survey. *Int. J. Environ. Res. Public Health* **2020**, *17*, 5598. [CrossRef] [PubMed]
15. Shihabi, S.; Al Nesser, S.; Hamadah, O. The preventive measures adopted during dental practice by the dentists in a low-income country to prevent the transmission of COVID-19: A questionnaire-based survey. *Indian J. Med Sci.* **2021**, *73*, 15–20. [CrossRef]
16. Pan, Y.; Liu, H.; Chu, C.; Li, X.; Liu, S.; Lu, S. Transmission Routes of SARS-CoV-2 and Protective Measures in Dental Clinics during the COVID-19 Pandemic. *Am. J. Dent.* **2020**, *33*, 129–134.
17. Moraes, R.R.; Correa, M.B.; Queiroz, A.B.; Daneris, Â.; Lopes, J.P.; Pereira-Cenci, T.; D'Avila, O.; Cenci, M.; Lima, G.D.S.; Demarco, F. COVID-19 challenges to dentistry in the new pandemic epicenter: Brazil. *PLoS ONE* **2020**, *15*, e0242251. [CrossRef]
18. Manuballa, S.; Abdelmaseh, M.; Tasgaonkar, N.; Frias, V.; Hess, M.; Crow, H.; Andreana, S.; Gupta, V.; Wooten, K.E.; Markiewicz, M.R.; et al. Managing the Oral Health of Cancer Patients during the COVID-19 Pandemic: Perspective of a Dental Clinic in a Cancer Center. *J. Clin. Med.* **2020**, *9*, 3138. [CrossRef]
19. Meng, L.; Hua, F.; Bian, Z. Coronavirus Disease 2019 (COVID-19): Emerging and Future Challenges for Dental and Oral Medicine. *J. Dent. Res.* **2020**, *99*, 481–487. [CrossRef]
20. Froum, S.H.; Froum, S.J. Incidence of COVID-19 Virus Transmission in Three Dental Offices: A 6-Month Retrospective Study. *Int. J. Periodontics Restor. Dent.* **2020**, *40*, 853–859. [CrossRef]
21. Hartig, M.; Stephens, C.; Foster, A.; Fontes, D.; Kinzel, M.; García-Godoy, F. Stopping the COVID-19 pandemic in dental offices: A review of SARS-CoV-2 transmission and cross-infection prevention. *Exp. Biol. Med.* **2021**, *246*, 2381–2390. [CrossRef] [PubMed]
22. Peng, X.; Xu, X.; Li, Y.; Cheng, L.; Zhou, X.; Ren, B. Transmission routes of 2019-nCoV and controls in dental practice. *Int. J. Oral Sci.* **2020**, *12*, 9. [CrossRef] [PubMed]
23. Araujo, M.W.B.; Estrich, C.G.; Mikkelsen, M.; Morrissey, R.; Harrison, B.; Geisinger, M.L.; Ioannidou, E.; Vujicic, M. COVID-2019 among Dentists in the United States: A 6-Month Longitudinal Report of Accumulative Prevalence and Incidence. *J. Am. Dent. Assoc.* **2021**, *152*, 425–433. [CrossRef] [PubMed]
24. Ge, Z.-Y.; Yang, L.-M.; Xia, J.-J.; Fu, X.-H.; Zhang, Y.-Z. Possible aerosol transmission of COVID-19 and special precautions in dentistry. *J. Zhejiang Univ. Sci. B* **2020**, *21*, 361–368. [CrossRef] [PubMed]
25. Dabiri, D.; Conti, S.R.; Pour, N.S.; Chong, A.; Dadjoo, S.; Dabiri, D.; Wiese, C.; Badal, J.; Hoogland, M.A.; Conti, H.R.; et al. A Multi-Disciplinary Review on the Aerobiology of COVID-19 in Dental Settings. *Front. Dent. Med.* **2021**, *2*, 66. [CrossRef] [PubMed]
26. Veeraiyan, D.N.; Varghese, S.S.; Rajasekar, A.; Karobari, M.I.; Thangavelu, L.; Marya, A.; Messina, P.; Scardina, G.A. Comparison of Interactive Teaching in Online and Offline Platforms among Dental Undergraduates. *Int. J. Environ. Res. Public Health* **2022**, *19*, 3170. [CrossRef]
27. Iqbal, A.; Ganji, K.K.; Khattak, O.; Shrivastava, D.; Srivastava, K.C.; Arjumand, B.; AlSharari, T.; A Alqahtani, A.M.; Hamza, M.O.; AbdelrahmanDafaalla, A.A.E.G. Enhancement of Skill Competencies in Operative Dentistry Using Procedure-Specific Educational Videos (E-Learning Tools) Post-COVID-19 Era—A Randomized Controlled Trial. *Int. J. Environ. Res. Public Health* **2022**, *19*, 4135. [CrossRef]
28. Fazio, M.; Lombardo, C.; Marino, G.; Marya, A.; Messina, P.; Scardina, G.A.; Tocco, A.; Torregrossa, F.; Valenti, C. LinguAPP: An m-Health Application for Teledentistry Diagnostics. *Int. J. Environ. Res. Public Health* **2022**, *19*, 822. [CrossRef]
29. Hamedani, S.; Farshidfar, N.; Ziaei, A.; Pakravan, H. The Dilemma of COVID-19 in Dental Practice Concerning the Role of Saliva in Transmission: A Brief Review of Current Evidence. *Eur. Oral Res.* **2020**, *54*, 92–100. [CrossRef]
30. Meethil, A.; Saraswat, S.; Chaudhary, P.; Dabdoub, S.; Kumar, P. Sources of SARS-CoV-2 and Other Microorganisms in Dental Aerosols. *J. Dent. Res.* **2021**, *100*, 817–823. [CrossRef]
31. Meister, T.L.; Brüggemann, Y.; Todt, D.; Conzelmann, C.; A Müller, J.; Groß, R.; Münch, J.; Krawczyk, A.; Steinmann, J.; Steinmann, J.; et al. Virucidal Efficacy of Different Oral Rinses against Severe Acute Respiratory Syndrome Coronavirus 2. *J. Infect. Dis.* **2020**, *222*, 1289–1292. [CrossRef] [PubMed]
32. Perry, E. How I Chose a Preprocedural Rinse—Registered Dental Hygienists. Available online: https://www.rdhmag.com/infection-control/article/14204889/how-i-chose-a-preprocedural-rinse (accessed on 15 December 2021).
33. Rutala, W.A.; Weber, D.J. *Guideline for Disinfection and Sterilization in Healthcare Facilities*; Centers for Disease Control and Prevention: Atlanta, GA, USA, 2008.
34. Ortega, K.L.; Rech, B.O.; el Haje, G.L.C.; Gallo, C.B.; Pérez-Sayáns, M.; Braz-Silva, P.H. Do Hydrogen Peroxide Mouthwashes Have a Virucidal Effect? A Systematic Review. *J. Hosp. Infect.* **2020**, *106*, 657–662. [CrossRef] [PubMed]
35. Don't Use Hydrogen Peroxide as a COVID-19 Pre-Procedural Rinse, Experts Say—Dental Tribune Canada. Available online: https://ca.dental-tribune.com/news/dont-use-hydrogen-peroxide-as-a-COVID-19-pre-procedural-rinse-experts-say/ (accessed on 15 December 2021).
36. Moskowitz, H.; Mendenhall, M. Comparative Analysis of Antiviral Efficacy of Four Different Mouthwashes against Severe Acute Respiratory Syndrome Coronavirus 2: An in Vitro Study. *Int. J. Exp. Dent. Sci.* **2020**, *9*, 1–3. [CrossRef]
37. Public Health Ontario. *Rapid Review: Open Operatory Dental Setting Infection Control Practices and Risk of Transmission during Aerosol-Generating Dental Procedures*; Public Health Ontario: Toronto, ON, Canada, 2020.

38. Steinhauer, K.; Meister, T.; Todt, D.; Krawczyk, A.; Paßvogel, L.; Becker, B.; Paulmann, D.; Bischoff, B.; Pfaender, S.; Brill, F.; et al. Comparison of the in-vitro efficacy of different mouthwash solutions targeting SARS-CoV-2 based on the European Standard EN 14476. *J. Hosp. Infect.* **2021**, *111*, 180–183. [CrossRef] [PubMed]
39. Oliveira, M.M.M.; De Almeida, A.C.; Rodrigues, C.M.d.C.; Sol, I.; Meneses-Santos, D. COVID-19—Mouthwash in dental clinical practice: Review. *Arch. Health Investig.* **2021**, *10*, 6–10. [CrossRef]
40. Mohd-Said, S.; Mohd-Dom, T.N.; Suhaimi, N.; Rani, H.; McGrath, C. Effectiveness of Pre-procedural Mouth Rinses in Reducing Aerosol Contamination During Periodontal Prophylaxis: A Systematic Review. *Front. Med.* **2021**, *8*, 600769. [CrossRef]
41. Kelly, N.; Nic Íomhair, A.; McKenna, G. Can oral rinses play a role in preventing transmission of COVID 19 infection? *Evid.-Based Dent.* **2020**, *21*, 42–43. [CrossRef]
42. Mohebbi, S.Z.; Ebrahimi, T.; Shamshiri, A.R. Do Mouthwashes Reduce COVID-19 Viral Load during Dental Procedures and Oropharyngeal Examinations? A Systematic Review. *Allergology* **2021**, *6*, 249. [CrossRef]
43. Butera, A.; Maiorani, C.; Natoli, V.; Bruni, A.; Coscione, C.; Magliano, G.; Giacobbo, G.; Morelli, A.; Moressa, S.; Scribante, A. Bio-Inspired Systems in Nonsurgical Periodontal Therapy to Reduce Contaminated Aerosol during COVID-19: A Comprehensive and Bibliometric Review. *J. Clin. Med.* **2020**, *9*, 3914. [CrossRef]
44. Farshidfar, N.; Jafarpour, D.; Hamedani, S.; Dziedzic, A.; Tanasiewicz, M. Proposal for Tier-Based Resumption of Dental Practice Determined by COVID-19 Rate, Testing and COVID-19 Vaccination: A Narrative Perspective. *J. Clin. Med.* **2021**, *10*, 2116. [CrossRef]
45. Shirazi, S.; Stanford, C.; Cooper, L. Characteristics and Detection Rate of SARS-CoV-2 in Alternative Sites and Specimens Pertaining to Dental Practice: An Evidence Summary. *J. Clin. Med.* **2021**, *10*, 1158. [CrossRef] [PubMed]
46. López-Verdín, S.; Prieto-Correa, J.R.; Molina-Frechero, N.; Bologna-Molina, R. Screening Test for COVID-19 in Dentai Practice: Best Options. *Am. J. Dent.* **2021**, *34*, 127–131. [PubMed]
47. Joshi, V.K. Dental treatment planning and management for the mouth cancer patient. *Oral Oncol.* **2010**, *46*, 475–479. [CrossRef] [PubMed]
48. Bertuzzi, A.F.; Ciccarelli, M.; Marrari, A.; Gennaro, N.; Dipasquale, A.; Giordano, L.; Cariboni, U.; Quagliuolo, V.L.; Alloisio, M.; Santoro, A. Impact of Active Cancer on COVID-19 Survival: A Matched-Analysis on 557 Consecutive Patients at an Academic Hospital in Lombardy, Italy. *Br. J. Cancer* **2021**, *125*, 358–365. [CrossRef]
49. Sinjari, B.; D'Ardes, D.; Santilli, M.; Rexhepi, I.; D'Addazio, G.; Di Carlo, P.; Chiacchiaretta, P.; Caputi, S.; Cipollone, F. SARS-CoV-2 and Oral Manifestation: An Observational, Human Study. *J. Clin. Med.* **2020**, *9*, 3218. [CrossRef]
50. dos Santos, J.A.; Normando, A.; da Silva, R.C.; Acevedo, A.; Canto, G.D.L.; Sugaya, N.; Santos-Silva, A.; Guerra, E. Oral Manifestations in Patients with COVID-19: A 6-Month Update. *J. Dent. Res.* **2021**, *100*, 1321–1329. [CrossRef]
51. Aragoneses, J.; Suárez, A.; Algar, J.; Rodríguez, C.; López-Valverde, N.; Aragoneses, J.M. Oral Manifestations of COVID-19: Updated Systematic Review With Meta-Analysis. *Front. Med.* **2021**, *8*, 1423. [CrossRef]
52. Orilisi, G.; Mascitti, M.; Togni, L.; Monterubbianesi, R.; Tosco, V.; Vitiello, F.; Santarelli, A.; Putignano, A.; Orsini, G. Oral Manifestations of COVID-19 in Hospitalized Patients: A Systematic Review. *Int. J. Environ. Res. Public Health* **2021**, *18*, 12511. [CrossRef]
53. Mekhemar, M.; Attia, S.; Dörfer, C.; Conrad, J. The Psychological Impact of the COVID-19 Pandemic on Dentists in Germany. *J. Clin. Med.* **2021**, *10*, 1008. [CrossRef]
54. Pylińska-Dąbrowska, D.; Starzyńska, A.; Cubała, W.J.; Ragin, K.; Alterio, D.; Jereczek-Fossa, B.A. Psychological Functioning of Patients Undergoing Oral Surgery Procedures during the Regime Related with SARS-CoV-2 Pandemic. *J. Clin. Med.* **2020**, *9*, 3344. [CrossRef]
55. Emodi-Perlman, A.; Eli, I.; Smardz, J.; Uziel, N.; Wieckiewicz, G.; Gilon, E.; Grychowska, N.; Wieckiewicz, M. Temporomandibular Disorders and Bruxism Outbreak as a Possible Factor of Orofacial Pain Worsening during the COVID-19 Pandemic—Concomitant Research in Two Countries. *J. Clin. Med.* **2020**, *9*, 3250. [CrossRef] [PubMed]
56. Olszewska, A.; Rzymski, P. Children's Dental Anxiety during the COVID-19 Pandemic: Polish Experience. *J. Clin. Med.* **2020**, *9*, 2751. [CrossRef] [PubMed]
57. Ahmadi, H.; Ebrahimi, A.; Ghorbani, F. The impact of COVID-19 pandemic on dental practice in Iran: A questionnaire-based report. *BMC Oral Health* **2020**, *20*, 354. [CrossRef] [PubMed]
58. Faccini, M.; Ferruzzi, F.; Mori, A.A.; Santin, G.C.; Oliveira, R.C.; de Oliveira, R.C.G.; Queiroz, P.M.; Salmeron, S.; Pini, N.I.P.; Sundfeld, D.; et al. Dental Care during COVID-19 Outbreak: A Web-Based Survey. *Eur. J. Dent.* **2020**, *14*, S14–S19. [CrossRef] [PubMed]
59. Basheer, S.N.; Vinothkumar, T.S.; Albar, N.H.M.; Karobari, M.I.; Renugalakshmi, A.; Bokhari, A.; Peeran, S.W.; Peeran, S.A.; Alhadri, L.M.; Tadakamadla, S.K. Knowledge of COVID-19 Infection Guidelines among the Dental Health Care Professionals of Jazan Region, Saudi Arabia. *Int. J. Environ. Res. Public Health* **2022**, *19*, 2034. [CrossRef] [PubMed]
60. Derruau, S.; Bouchet, J.; Nassif, A.; Baudet, A.; Yasukawa, K.; Lorimier, S.; Prêcheur, I.; Bloch-Zupan, A.; Pellat, B.; Chardin, H.; et al. COVID-19 and Dentistry in 72 Questions: An Overview of the Literature. *J. Clin. Med.* **2021**, *10*, 779. [CrossRef]
61. Cagetti, M.G.; Cairoli, J.L.; Senna, A. Guglielmo Campus COVID-19 Outbreak in North Italy: An Overview on Dentistry. A Questionnaire Survey. *Int. J. Environ. Res. Public Health* **2020**, *17*, 3835. [CrossRef]
62. Sfikas, P.M. Teledentistry: Legal and Regulatory Issues Explored. *J. Am. Dent. Assoc.* **1997**, *128*, 1716–1718. [CrossRef]

63. Kravitz, N.D.; Burris, B.; Butler, D.; Dabney, C.W. Teledentistry, Do-It-Yourself Orthodontics, and Remote Treatment Monitoring. *J. Clin. Orthod.* **2016**, *50*, 718–726.
64. Park, J.H.; Rogowski, L.; Kim, J.H.; Al Shami, S.; Howell, S.E.I. Teledentistry Platforms for Orthodontics. *J. Clin. Pediatr. Dent.* **2021**, *45*, 48–53. [CrossRef]
65. A Mandall, N.; O'Brien, K.; Brady, J.; Worthington, H.; Harvey, L. Teledentistry for screening new patient orthodontic referrals. Part 1: A randomised controlled trial. *Br. Dent. J.* **2005**, *199*, 659–662. [CrossRef] [PubMed]
66. Giudice, A.; Barone, S.; Muraca, D.; Averta, F.; Diodati, F.; Antonelli, A.; Fortunato, L. Can Teledentistry Improve the Monitoring of Patients during the COVID-19 Dissemination? A Descriptive Pilot Study. *Int. J. Environ. Res. Public Health* **2020**, *17*, 3399. [CrossRef] [PubMed]
67. Maspero, C.; Abate, A.; Cavagnetto, D.; El Morsi, M.; Fama, A.; Farronato, M. Available Technologies, Applications and Benefits of Teleorthodontics. A Literature Review and Possible Applications during the COVID-19 Pandemic. *J. Clin. Med.* **2020**, *9*, 1891. [CrossRef] [PubMed]
68. Deana, N.F.; Seiffert, A.; Aravena-Rivas, Y.; Alonso-Coello, P.; Muñoz-Millán, P.; Espinoza-Espinoza, G.; Pineda, P.; Zaror, C. Recommendations for Safe Dental Care: A Systematic Review of Clinical Practice Guidelines in the First Year of the COVID-19 Pandemic. *Int. J. Environ. Res. Public Health* **2021**, *18*, 10059. [CrossRef]
69. Statement on Omicron Sublineage BA.2. Available online: https://www.who.int/news/item/22-02-2022-statement-on-omicron-sublineage-ba.2 (accessed on 18 March 2022).
70. Hoyte, T.; Kowlessar, A.; Mahabir, A.; Khemkaran, K.; Jagroo, P.; Jahoor, S. The Knowledge, Awareness, and Attitude Regarding COVID-19 among Trinidad and Tobago Dentists. A Cross-Sectional Survey. *Oral* **2021**, *1*, 250–260. [CrossRef]
71. Estrich, C.G.; Mikkelsen, M.; Morrissey, R.; Geisinger, M.L.; Ioannidou, E.; Vujicic, M.; Araujo, M.W.B. Estimating COVID-19 prevalence and infection control practices among US dentists. *J. Am. Dent. Assoc.* **2020**, *151*, 815–824. [CrossRef]
72. Gugnani, N.; Gugnani, S. Safety protocols for dental practices in the COVID-19 era. *Evid.-Based Dent.* **2020**, *21*, 56–57. [CrossRef]
73. Souza, A.F.; de Arruda, J.A.A.; Costa, F.P.D.; Bemquerer, L.M.; Castro, W.H.; Campos, F.E.B.; Kakehasi, F.M.; Travassos, D.V.; Silva, T.A. Safety protocols for dental care during the COVID-19 pandemic: The experience of a Brazilian hospital service. *Braz. Oral Res.* **2021**, *35*, e070. [CrossRef]
74. Bizzoca, M.E.; Campisi, G.; Muzio, L.L. An innovative risk-scoring system of dental procedures and safety protocols in the COVID-19 era. *BMC Oral Health* **2020**, *20*, 1–8. [CrossRef]
75. Alsaegh, A.; Belova, E.; Vasil'Ev, Y.; Zabroda, N.; Severova, L.; Timofeeva, M.; Dobrokhotov, D.; Leonova, A.; Mitrokhin, O. COVID-19 in Dental Settings: Novel Risk Assessment Approach. *Int. J. Environ. Res. Public Health* **2021**, *18*, 6093. [CrossRef]
76. Falahchai, M.; Hemmati, Y.B.; Hasanzade, M. Dental care management during the COVID-19 outbreak. *Spéc. Care Dent.* **2020**, *40*, 539–548. [CrossRef] [PubMed]
77. Attia, S.; Howaldt, H.-P. Impact of COVID-19 on the Dental Community: Part I before Vaccine (BV). *J. Clin. Med.* **2021**, *10*, 288. [CrossRef] [PubMed]
78. Riad, A.; Pokorná, A.; Attia, S.; Klugarová, J.; Koščík, M.; Klugar, M. Prevalence of COVID-19 Vaccine Side Effects among Healthcare Workers in the Czech Republic. *J. Clin. Med.* **2021**, *10*, 1428. [CrossRef]
79. Chen, J.; Wang, R.; Gilby, N.B.; Wei, G.-W. Omicron (B.1.1.529): Infectivity, Vaccine Breakthrough, and Antibody Resistance. *arXiv* **2021**, arXiv:2112.01318. [CrossRef] [PubMed]
80. Cele, S.; Jackson, L.; Khan, K.; Khoury, D.; Moyo-Gwete, T.; Tegally, H.; Scheepers, C.; Amoako, D.; Karim, F.; Bernstein, M.; et al. SARS-CoV-2 Omicron Has Extensive but Incomplete Escape of Pfizer BNT162b2 Elicited Neutralization and Requires ACE2 for Infection. *medRxiv* **2021**. [CrossRef]
81. Wilhelm, A.; Widera, M.; Grikscheit, K.; Toptan, T.; Schenk, B.; Pallas, C.; Metzler, M.; Kohmer, N.; Hoehl, S.; Helfritz, F.A.; et al. Reduced Neutralization of SARS-CoV-2 Omicron Variant by Vaccine Sera and Monoclonal Antibodies. *medRxiv* **2021**. [CrossRef]
82. Gruell, H.; Vanshylla, K. MRNA Booster Immunization Elicits Potent Neutralizing Serum Activity against the SARS-CoV-2 Omicron Variant. Available online: https://drive.google.com/file/d/13iHMR6rk3MKRFhDZmNuH3AAjR1uT8mEU/view (accessed on 15 December 2021).
83. HKUMed Finds Omicron SARS-CoV-2 Can Infect Faster and Better than Delta in Human Bronchus but with Less Severe Infection in Lung—News—HKUMed. Available online: http://www.med.hku.hk/en/news/press/20211215-omicron-SARS-COV-2-infection (accessed on 15 December 2021).
84. Cameroni, E.; Saliba, C.; Bowen, J.E.; Rosen, L.E.; Culap, K.; Pinto, D.; de Marco, A.; Zepeda, S.K.; di Iulio, J.; Zatta, F.; et al. Broadly Neutralizing Antibodies Overcome SARS-CoV-2 Omicron Antigenic Shift. *bioRxiv* **2021**. [CrossRef] [PubMed]
85. Enhancing Readiness for Omicron (B.1.1.529): Technical Brief and Priority Actions for Member States. Available online: https://www.who.int/publications/m/item/enhancing-readiness-for-omicron-(b.1.1.529)-technical-brief-and-priority-actions-for-member-states (accessed on 15 December 2021).
86. Yamasoba, D.; Kimura, I.; Nasser, H.; Morioka, Y.; Nao, N.; Ito, J.; Uriu, K.; Tsuda, M.; Zahradnik, J.; Shirakawa, K.; et al. Virological Characteristics of SARS-CoV-2 BA.2 Variant. *bioRxiv* **2022**. [CrossRef]
87. Classification of Omicron (B.1.1.529): SARS-CoV-2 Variant of Concern. Available online: https://www.who.int/news/item/26-11-2021-classification-of-omicron-(b.1.1.529)-sars-cov-2-variant-of-concern (accessed on 12 December 2021).

88. Moderna—Moderna Announces Strategy to Address Omicron (B.1.1.529) SARS-CoV-2 Variant. Available online: https://investors.modernatx.com/news/news-details/2021/Moderna-Announces-Strategy-to-Address-Omicron-B.1.1.529-SARS-CoV-2-Variant/default.aspx (accessed on 12 December 2021).
89. Karim, S.S.A.; Karim, Q.A. Omicron SARS-CoV-2 Variant: A New Chapter in the COVID-19 Pandemic. *Lancet* **2021**, *398*, 2126–2128. [CrossRef]
90. Pulliam, J.R.C.; van Schalkwyk, C.; Govender, N.; von Gottberg, A.; Cohen, C.; Groome, M.J.; Dushoff, J.; Mlisana, K.; Moultrie, H. Increased risk of SARS-CoV-2 reinfection associated with emergence of the Omicron variant in South Africa. *medrxiv* **2021**. [CrossRef]
91. Van Kasteren, P.B.; van Der Veer, B.; van den Brink, S.; Wijsman, L.; de Jonge, J.; van den Brandt, A.; Molenkamp, R.; Reusken, C.B.E.M.; Meijer, A. Comparison of seven commercial RT-PCR diagnostic kits for COVID-19. *J. Clin. Virol.* **2020**, *128*, 104412. [CrossRef] [PubMed]
92. Mushtaq, M.Z.; Shakoor, S.; Kanji, A.; Shaheen, N.; Nasir, A.; Ansar, Z.; Ahmed, I.; Mahmood, S.F.; Hasan, R.; Hasan, Z. Discrepancy between PCR Based SARS-CoV-2 Tests Suggests the Need to Re-Evaluate Diagnostic Assays. *BMC Res. Notes* **2021**, *14*, 316. [CrossRef] [PubMed]
93. Planas, D.; Saunders, N.; Maes, P.; Guivel-Benhassine, F.; Planchais, C.; Buchrieser, J.; Bolland, W.-H.; Porrot, F.; Staropoli, I.; Lemoine, F.; et al. Considerable Escape of SARS-CoV-2 Variant Omicron to Antibody Neutralization. *bioRxiv* **2021**. [CrossRef]
94. Brandal, L.T.; MacDonald, E.; Veneti, L.; Ravlo, T.; Lange, H.; Naseer, U.; Feruglio, S.; Bragstad, K.; Hungnes, O.; Ødeskaug, L.E.; et al. Outbreak Caused by the SARS-CoV-2 Omicron Variant in Norway, November to December 2021. *Euro Surveill. Bull. Eur. Sur Les Mal. Transm. Eur. Commun. Dis. Bull.* **2021**, *26*, 2101147. [CrossRef] [PubMed]
95. Kuhlmann, C.; Mayer, C.K.; Claassen, M.; Maponga, T.G.; Sutherland, A.D.; Suliman, T.; Shaw, M.; Preiser, W. Breakthrough Infections with SARS-CoV-2 Omicron Variant Despite Booster Dose of MRNA Vaccine. *SSRN Electron. J.* **2021**. [CrossRef]
96. Ahmed, S.F.; Quadeer, A.A.; McKay, M.R. SARS-CoV-2 T Cell Responses Elicited by COVID-19 Vaccines or Infection Are Expected to Remain Robust against Omicron. *Viruses* **2022**, *14*, 79. [CrossRef]
97. SARS-CoV-2 Variants of Concern as of 13 January 2022. Available online: https://www.ecdc.europa.eu/en/covid-19/variants-concern (accessed on 14 January 2022).
98. Volgenant, C.M.C.; de Soet, J.J. Cross-transmission in the Dental Office: Does This Make You Ill? *Curr. Oral Health Rep.* **2018**, *5*, 221–228. [CrossRef]
99. Nemati, S. Impacts of COVID-19 Outbreak on Dentistry Dimensions. *Indian J. Med Sci.* **2021**, *46*, 149–150. [CrossRef]
100. Higgins, V.; Sohaei, D.; Diamandis, E.P.; Prassas, I. COVID-19: From an acute to chronic disease? Potential long-term health consequences. *Crit. Rev. Clin. Lab. Sci.* **2020**, *58*, 297–310. [CrossRef]
101. McDonald, L.T. Healing after COVID-19: Are survivors at risk for pulmonary fibrosis? *Am. J. Physiol. Cell. Mol. Physiol.* **2021**, *320*, L257–L265. [CrossRef]
102. Mishra, S.K.; Tripathi, T. One Year Update on the COVID-19 Pandemic: Where Are We Now? *Acta Trop.* **2021**, *214*, 105778. [CrossRef] [PubMed]
103. Baig, A.M. Deleterious Outcomes in Long-Hauler COVID-19: The Effects of SARS-CoV-2 on the CNS in Chronic COVID Syndrome. *ACS Chem. Neurosci.* **2020**, *11*, 4017–4020. [CrossRef] [PubMed]
104. Valenzano, A.; Scarinci, A.; Monda, V.; Sessa, F.; Messina, A.; Monda, M.; Precenzano, F.; Mollica, M.; Carotenuto, M.; Messina, G.; et al. The Social Brain and Emotional Contagion: COVID-19 Effects. *Medicina* **2020**, *56*, 640. [CrossRef] [PubMed]
105. Evans, P.C.; Rainger, G.E.; Mason, J.C.; Guzik, T.J.; Osto, E.; Stamataki, Z.; Neil, D.; Hoefer, I.E.; Fragiadaki, M.; Waltenberger, J.; et al. Endothelial dysfunction in COVID-19: A position paper of the ESC Working Group for Atherosclerosis and Vascular Biology, and the ESC Council of Basic Cardiovascular Science. *Cardiovasc. Res.* **2020**, *116*, 2177–2184. [CrossRef] [PubMed]
106. Madjunkov, M.; Dviri, M.; Librach, C. A comprehensive review of the impact of COVID-19 on human reproductive biology, assisted reproduction care and pregnancy: A Canadian perspective. *J. Ovarian Res.* **2020**, *13*, 1–18. [CrossRef]
107. Wang, N.; Qin, L.; Ma, L.; Yan, H. Effect of severe acute respiratory syndrome coronavirus-2 (SARS-CoV-2) on reproductive system. *Stem Cell Res.* **2021**, *52*, 102189. [CrossRef]
108. Thurzo, A.; Kočiš, F.; Novák, B.; Czako, L.; Varga, I. Three-Dimensional Modeling and 3D Printing of Biocompatible Orthodontic Power-Arm Design with Clinical Application. *Appl. Sci.* **2021**, *11*, 9693. [CrossRef]
109. Thurzo, A.; Urbanová, W.; Novák, B.; Waczulíková, I.; Varga, I. Utilization of a 3D Printed Orthodontic Distalizer for Tooth-Borne Hybrid Treatment in Class II Unilateral Malocclusions. *Materials* **2022**, *15*, 1740. [CrossRef]
110. Takanabe, Y.; Maruoka, Y.; Kondo, J.; Yagi, S.; Chikazu, D.; Okamoto, R.; Saitoh, M. Dispersion of Aerosols Generated during Dental Therapy. *Int. J. Environ. Res. Public Health* **2021**, *18*, 11279. [CrossRef]
111. Rexhepi, I.; Mangifesta, R.; Santilli, M.; Guri, S.; Di Carlo, P.; D'Addazio, G.; Caputi, S.; Sinjari, B. Effects of Natural Ventilation and Saliva Standard Ejectors during the COVID-19 Pandemic: A Quantitative Analysis of Aerosol Produced during Dental Procedures. *Int. J. Environ. Res. Public Health* **2021**, *18*, 7472. [CrossRef]
112. Herishanu, Y.; Avivi, I.; Aharon, A.; Shefer, G.; Levi, S.; Bronstein, Y.; Morales, M.; Ziv-Baran, T.; Arbel, Y.S.; Scarfò, L.; et al. Efficacy of the BNT162b2 mRNA COVID-19 vaccine in patients with chronic lymphocytic leukemia. *Blood* **2021**, *137*, 3165–3173. [CrossRef] [PubMed]

113. WHO Director-General's Opening Remarks at the Media Briefing on COVID-19—14 December 2021. Available online: https://www.who.int/director-general/speeches/detail/who-director-general-s-opening-remarks-at-the-media-briefing-on-covid-19---14-december-2021 (accessed on 16 December 2021).
114. Bjornevik, K.; Cortese, M.; Healy, B.C.; Kuhle, J.; Mina, M.J.; Leng, Y.; Elledge, S.J.; Niebuhr, D.W.; Scher, A.I.; Munger, K.L.; et al. Longitudinal analysis reveals high prevalence of Epstein-Barr virus associated with multiple sclerosis. *Science* **2022**, *375*, 296–301. [CrossRef] [PubMed]
115. Wang, L.; Berger, N.A.; Kaelber, D.C.; Davis, P.B.; Volkow, N.D.; Xu, R. Comparison of Outcomes from COVID Infection in Pediatric and Adult Patients before and after the Emergence of Omicron. *medRxiv* **2022**. [CrossRef]

International Journal of
Environmental Research and Public Health

MDPI

Article

Enhancement of Skill Competencies in Operative Dentistry Using Procedure-Specific Educational Videos (E-Learning Tools) Post-COVID-19 Era—A Randomized Controlled Trial

Azhar Iqbal [1,2], Kiran Kumar Ganji [3,4,*], Osama Khattak [1], Deepti Shrivastava [3], Kumar Chandan Srivastava [5], Bilal Arjumand [6], Thani AlSharari [7], Ali Mosfer A Alqahtani [8], May Othman Hamza [9] and Ahmed Abu El Gasim AbdelrahmanDafaalla [10]

1 Department of Operative Dentistry & Endodontics, College of Dentistry, Jouf University, Sakaka 72345, Saudi Arabia; dr.azhar.iqbal@jodent.org; dr.osama.khattak@jodent.org
2 Department of Operative Dentistry & Endodontics, Frontier Medical and Dental College, Abbottabad 22010, Pakistan
3 Department of Preventive Dentistry, College of Dentistry, Jouf University, Sakaka 72345, Saudi Arabia; sdeepti20@gmail.com
4 Department of Periodontics, Sharad Pawar Dental College & Hospital, Datta Meghe Insitute of Medical Sciences, Nagpur 440016, India
5 Department of Oral & Maxillofacial Surgery and Diagnostic Sciences, College of Dentistry, Jouf University, Sakaka 72345, Saudi Arabia; drkcs.omr@gmail.com
6 Department of Conservative Dental Sciences and Endodontics, College of Dentistry, Qassim University, Qassim 52571, Saudi Arabia; ba.ahmad@qu.edu.sa
7 Restorative and Dental Materials Department, Faculty of Dentistry, Taif University, Taif 26571, Saudi Arabia; thani.alsharari@gmail.com
8 Department of Diagnostic Dental Sciences, College of Dentistry, King Khalid University, Abha 62529, Saudi Arabia; al.alqahtani@kku.edu.sa
9 Department of Prosthetic Dental Sciences, College of Dentistry, Jouf University, Sakaka 72345, Saudi Arabia; dr.may.hamza@jodent.org
10 Department of Urology, King Abdulaziz Specialist Hospital, Sakaka 72345, Saudi Arabia; yazangasim@gmail.com
* Correspondence: kiranperio@gmail.com

Citation: Iqbal, A.; Ganji, K.K.; Khattak, O.; Shrivastava, D.; Srivastava, K.C.; Arjumand, B.; AlSharari, T.; Alqahtani, A.M.A.; Hamza, M.O.; AbdelrahmanDafaalla, A.A.E.G. Enhancement of Skill Competencies in Operative Dentistry Using Procedure-Specific Educational Videos (E-Learning Tools) Post-COVID-19 Era—A Randomized Controlled Trial. *Int. J. Environ. Res. Public Health* **2022**, *19*, 4135. https://doi.org/10.3390/ijerph19074135

Academic Editors: Giuseppe Alessandro Scardina, Giorgio Rappelli and Paul B. Tchounwou

Received: 6 February 2022
Accepted: 28 March 2022
Published: 31 March 2022

Abstract: E-learning has completely transformed how people teach and learn, particularly in the last three pandemic years. This study evaluated the effectiveness of additional procedure-specific video demonstrations through E-learning in improving the knowledge and practical preclinical skills acquisition of undergraduate dental students in comparison with live demonstration only. A randomized controlled trial was conducted for the second-year dental students in the College of Dentistry, Jouf University, to evaluate the impact of E-learning-assisted videos on preclinical skill competency levels in operative dentistry. After a brief introduction to this study, the second-year male and female students voluntarily participated in the survey through an official college email. Fifty participants were enrolled in the study after obtaining informed consent. The participants were randomly divided into two groups, twenty-five each. The control group (Group A) was taught using traditional methods, and the intervention group (Group B) used E-learning-assisted educational videos and traditional techniques. An objective structured practical examination (OSPE) was used to assess both groups. The faculty members prepared a structured, standardized form to evaluate students. After OSPE, statistical analysis was done to compare the grades of OSPE between Group A and Group B. Logistic regression analysis was done to express the effect of components of the OSPE on gender, cumulative gross point average (CGPA), Group A and Group B. The results showed a significant difference in the experimental groups after the intervention ($p < 0.000$). The simulator position parameter demonstrated that the participants had a significant competence level after the intervention by procedure-specific videos ($p < 0.000$) and an exponential value of 6.494. The participants taught by E-learning-assisted procedure-specific videos and traditional teaching strategies demonstrated an enhanced learning and skill competency level than participants who used only traditional teaching strategies.

Keywords: dental skills; operative dentistry; procedure-specific videos; E-learning; dental education

1. Introduction

The undergraduate dental program concentrates on the students' psychomotor skill development throughout their early preclinical years, often notably applicable to the preclinical operative courses in the dentistry curriculum. The students are exposed to the technical aspects of practical preclinical skills, which play a vital role in boosting the outcome of clinical procedures [1]. Usually, the dental faculties use a standard, traditional live demonstration methodology for teaching preclinical laboratory skills. The live demonstration in small clusters has been helpful in teaching the preclinical laboratory skills due to its improved communication skills and accumulated student confidence, and provided a higher understanding of the procedure than informative, didactic teaching [2,3]. However, various studies have shown that the live demonstration–based teaching methodology has several drawbacks, such as difficulty in the visualization of the procedure, the reliance on the students on the instructor, and slight variations of the procedure among the different instructors [2–4]. Aside from these drawbacks, the live demonstrations' effectiveness depends on the number of students allotted to the instructor and the amount of time spent delivering the live demonstration. Another issue associated with the live demonstration is, it is delivered only once for a particular selected procedure. Therefore, students might not get an opportunity to repeatedly follow the procedure to understand and master the essential skills. According to one study, the traditional teaching methodology has caused significant psychological distress, which results in anxiety, depression and burnout among the students [2]. Due to the present situation of the COVID-19 pandemic, the students and faculty had to follow social distancing norms that made it even worse for the students to visualize the procedure properly. Keeping in view these drawbacks of traditional teaching methodologies, and conjointly because of the technological advancement in the past few decades [5–8], it has become essential for educators and clinicians to bring their teaching styles and methodology in line with the current pandemic situation and the students' learning needs and training desires to reinforce and improve their knowledge and preclinical and clinical skill competency [9–12]. There is a place for vicarious and experiential learning strategies in clinical skills training. Clinical teachers must use learner-centered ways to get to know their students, as well as their students' strengths, limitations, talents and experiences [13]. Therefore, educators and clinicians are trying to find new teaching methodologies for preclinical laboratory skills. Procedure-specific educational videos and video demonstrations could be blended and integrated with preclinical live demonstrations. These procedure-specific educational videos permit students to visualize the procedural steps within the lab on the projector and E-learning tools on Blackboard, on-campus and off-campus [14]. This will allow the students to revise the procedural steps before, during, and after the skill lab session as per the students' convenience [15]. It also reduces information differences and bias and provides uniformity in learning experiences for all students [2]. Since we have entered a digital era, the concept of E-learning in various forms has emerged as an effective tool for teaching strategies [16]. E-learning can be defined as learning while utilizing electronic technologies to access educational curricula outside a traditional classroom [17,18]. Video demonstration through one of the E-learning tools, such as Blackboard has been witnessed as an implicit tool. Literature suggests that students are more inclined toward the newer teaching method than traditional learning [19]. Recently, Elham Soltanimehr discovered that virtual learning is better than traditional lecture-based learning for knowledge acquisition augmentation during the diagnostic imaging of bone lesions of the jaw [20]. Therefore, he has suggested that virtual educational programs must be revised to improve the student's reporting skills [20]. Kon H et al. showed in their study that the videotapes were considered valuable resources because a better visualization of the procedure can be achieved by repeated replay and review functions. Hence, videotapes were considered a useful and valuable recap tool for the clinical demonstration during denture construction [21]. Wong et al., in their study, showed that the use of instructional videos has been found effective in complementing the advanced trauma life support approach for teaching psychomotor skills in the administration of local anesthetics by oral health students [19]. Due to the present pandemic situation of COVID-19 and the lack of or limited in-campus teaching due to social distancing restrictions, we were compelled to enhance students' knowledge and skills by utilizing the support of E-learning. This study hypothesized whether the addition of procedure-specific video demonstrations (E-learning) improves the acquisition of knowledge and preclinical practical skills for undergraduate dental students in comparison with live demonstrations only.

2. Methods

Male and female second-year dental students from the College of Dentistry, Jouf University, who passed their prerequisite courses for the preclinical operative dentistry skill course, were recruited for the study voluntarily after signing an informed consent form. The dental undergraduate students with any psychomotor disability were excluded from the study. The study was conducted during the scheduled laboratory hours in the college premises after ethical approval was taken from the local bioethics committee with no 254-1-2020, as per institutional policy. Using computer-generated random numbers, these participants were randomly divided into the control group (Group A) and the experimental group (Group B), using simple randomization sampling based on teaching methodology ($n = 25$). Sample size calculation was done by using the G*Power computing tool (Heinrich-Heine-Universität Düsseldorf, Germany), a confidence interval (α) of 0.05 and power ($1 - \beta$) 95–0.95%, the difference between the two dependent means (matched pairs) and effect size (f) of 0.5. The total sample size generated was found to be five; however, four students were unable to participate in the study due to some personal reasons. The skill-based procedure under evaluation was a part of the preclinical second-year dental undergraduate curriculum.

The participants in the control group (Group A) were taught about the skill-based procedure with the routine live lab demonstration. Contrarily, the participants in the experimental group (Group B) were taught by using a procedure-specific educational video demonstration through an E-learning tool (Blackboard) plus the routine live lab demonstration, described as a hybrid (Figure 1). The live demonstration and procedure-specific educational video described the identical steps for the class I cavity preparation and amalgam restoration on typodont tooth no. 36. The procedure involved 330 carbide burs in a high-speed handpiece with air–water spray, a mouth mirror, explorer and periodontal probe. The live demonstration was given by an experienced academician who handled preclinical and clinical work. The procedure-specific educational video was also produced by the same faculty member who gave the live demonstration to avoid any information differences regarding the procedure.

On the day of the live demonstration, the procedure-specific video was sent through Blackboard to the experimental group (Group B) participants who were instructed by a Blackboard announcement and official institutional email to watch the procedural-specific videos before attending the evaluation session for the same procedure in the next scheduled lab hours for both groups. A request was made to the institutional E-learning unit that access should not be provided to the control group (Group A) participants. The video could not be recorded or copied by the experimental group (Group B) participants to avoid sharing it with the control group (Group A) participants. Statistical tracking through Blackboard was enabled to ensure that participants viewed the video for a minimum of five to six views. After one week, an objective structured practical examination (OSPE) was conducted for both groups to assess the clinical competency level of achievement resulting from this intervention. The OSPE consisted of six stations: infection control and operator position, tray organization, simulator position, cavity outline and extension, resistance form and retention form, which were considered outcome variables. To maintain the inter-examiner reliability, Cohen's kappa statistic was used to measure the agreement level between the scores of the OSPE assessed by two faculty members who were not involved in any of the steps of this study. The kappa score between the two faculty members was found to be 0.88. The participants of both groups were anonymized by the examiners. The average score of the two examiners was taken as the score of that OSPE station. The final average scores of all the OSPE stations were calculated, but these did not contribute to the student's midterm or final term exam grades. It was made sure by the course organizer that the examiners did not share the result. At the end of the study, a questionnaire containing seven questions was circulated among the students to get their feedback, assess their perception of the teaching methodologies, and compare them.

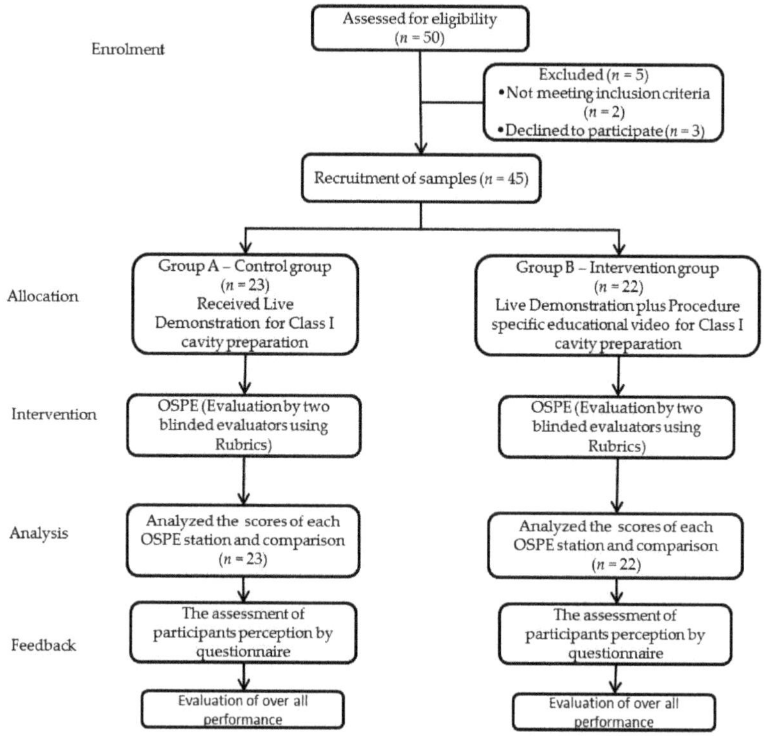

Figure 1. Summary of research methodology and experimental protocol.

Statistical Analyses

After any necessary editing, the biographic and assessment sheet data were transferred into an Excel sheet. The participant's personal information was treated anonymously for their privacy and confidentiality; therefore, a code/sequence was given to each subject for identification. The descriptive analysis (presentation of data in the form of percentage and mean with standard deviation) and inferential analysis, such as the McNemar test were used to assess the test of significance related to competent and non-competent between the control and experimental groups, and logistic regression analysis was done to express the effect of OSPE performances on gender, CGPA, control and experimental group, using a statistical package for the social sciences (SPSS IBM, version 21, Chicago, IL, USA).

3. Results

There were 50 participants, 28 males (56%) and 22 females (44%), in this study. These participants were randomly divided into two groups: control and experimental. There were 25 participants in each group (n = 25), 14 males (56%) and 11 females (44%). The results

(Table 1) show that there was no significant difference before the intervention between the control group and the experimental group in the competence level of the participants, but a significant difference was found in the experimental groups (Table 2) after the intervention. The p value was 0.000. Among all the study variables, only a simulator position has shown that the participants had a significant competence level after the intervention by procedure-specific videos, with a p value of 0.000 and an exponential value of 6.494.

Table 1. McNemar test analysis for competent and non-competent in the control group.

2 × 2 Contingency Table for Control Group (Before & After)					
		Control Group After		**Total**	***p*-Value**
		Non-Competent	**Competent**		
Control group before	Non-competent	122	0	122	0.352
	Competent	12	41	53	
Total		134	41	175	

Table 2. McNemar test analysis for competent and non-competent in the experimental group.

2 × 2 Contingency Table for Experimental Group (Before & After)					
		Experimental Group After		**Total**	***p*-Value**
		Non-Competent	**Competent**		
Experimental group before	Non-competent	34	0	34	0.000
	Competent	22	119	141	
Total		56	119	175	

Binomial logistic regression was performed to ascertain the effects of infection control, operator position, tray organization, simulator position, cavity outline and extension, resistance form and retention form parameters on the likelihood that participants were successful in the skilled procedure. The percentage of variance in being competent within the measured parameters, such as for infection control was 52.3%, operator position 54%, tray organization 60%, simulator position 45%, cavity outline and extension 61%, resistance form 65%, and retention form 65 %.

The effect of the infection control parameter on the students' competence level demonstrated a significant difference between males and females (p value, 0.000; odds ratio, 40.3) in which females were considered constant. Under the CGPA group, there was a significant difference with different levels of CGPA score (p value, 0.000; odds ratio, 325). Finally, concerning infection control, there was a significant difference among groups 1, 2, and 3 (p value, 0.000). The effect of operator position on the students' competency level demonstrated a significant difference between male and female groups (p value, 0.001; odds ratio, 40.389). Regarding the CGPA group, there was a significant difference with different levels of CGPA score (p value, 0.000; odds ratio, 325.42). There was no significant difference found among groups 1, 2, and 3 regarding the operator position. Regarding the tray organization, a significant difference was found regarding CGPA level (p value, 0.003; odds ratio, 25.916) according to the binary logistic regression analysis results. Regarding the genders and among different groups, no significant difference was found. Regarding the cavity preparation outline and extension, a significant difference was found (p value, 0.004; odds ratio, 0.044) in group 3 among the different groups. A significant difference was found (p value, 0.003; odds ratio, 51.010) among the different CGPA levels during the binary logistic regression analysis (Tables 3–7).

Table 3. Expressing the effect of infection control and operator position parameters on gender, CGPA, Group A and Group B using binary logistic regression analysis.

Parameter	Variables	B	S.E.	Wald	df	Sig.	Exp (B)	95% C.I. for EXP (B)	
								Lower	Upper
Infection control & Operator position	Gender	3.69	1.10	11.17	1	0.001	4.38	4.62	5.097
	CGPA	5.7	1.47	15.448	1	0.000	5.25	18.17	5.25
	Group A	0.66	0.82	0.644	1	0.422	1.93	0.38	9.68
	Group B	1.2	0.72	2.78	1	0.095	3.32	0.81	13.65
	Constant	−26.99	6.94	15.11	1	0.000	0.000		

Table 4. Expressing the effect of tray organization parameter on gender, CGPA, Group A and Group B using binary logistic regression analysis.

Parameter	Variables	B	S.E.	Wald	df	Sig.	Exp (B)	95% C.I. for EXP (B)	
								Lower	Upper
Tray Organization	Gender	0.80	1.05	0.58	1	0.445	2.23	0.28	3.68
	CGPA	3.25	1.10	8.72	1	0.003	25.91	2.98	3.45
	Group A	−1.33	0.84	2.47	1	0.115	0.26	0.05	1.38
	Group B	1.08	0.88	1.48	1	0.223	2.94	0.51	2.76
	Constant	−13.14	5.24	6.28	1	0.012	0.00		

Table 5. Expressing the effect of simulator position parameter on gender, CGPA, Group A and Group B using binary logistic regression analysis.

Parameter	Variables	B	S.E.	Wald	df	Sig.	Exp (B)	95% C.I. for EXP (B)	
								Lower	Upper
Simulator position	Gender	1.87	0.92	4.13	1	0.042	6.49	1.06	6.46
	CGPA	2.41	0.89	7.20	1	0.007	11.17	1.91	65.11
	Group A	−1.68	0.75	5.04	1	0.025	0.18	0.04	0.80
	Group B	0.00	0.69	0.00	1	1.000	1.00	0.25	3.92
	Constant	−10.15	4.24	5.71	1	0.017	0.00		

Table 6. Expressing the effect of cavity outline and extension parameter on gender, CGPA, Group A and Group B using binary logistic regression analysis.

Parameter	Variables	B	S.E.	Wald	df	Sig.	Exp (B)	95% C.I. for EXP (B)	
								Lower	Upper
Cavity outline and extension	Gender	−1.65	1.18	1.93	1	0.164	0.19	0.01	1.96
	CGPA	1.72	0.99	3.04	1	0.081	5.62	0.80	3.14
	Group A	−2.15	1.02	4.40	1	0.036	0.11	0.01	0.86
	Group B	0.33	0.82	0.16	1	0.684	1.39	0.28	6.97
	Constant	−4.60	4.89	0.88	1	0.347	0.01		

Table 7. Expressing the effect of resistance form and retention form parameter on gender, CGPA, Group A and Group B using binary logistic regression analysis.

Parameter	Variables	B	S.E.	Wald	df	Sig.	Exp (B)	95% C.I. for EXP (B)	
								Lower	Upper
Resistance form & Retention form	Gender	0.04	1.09	0.00	1	0.965	1.04	0.12	8.89
	CGPA	3.93	1.31	8.98	1	0.003	11.01	3.89	5.36
	Group A	−0.23	0.93	0.06	1	0.804	0.79	0.126	4.99
	Group B	2.09	0.95	4.83	1	0.028	8.09	1.25	3.57
	Constant	−16.28	6.20	6.88	1	0.009	0.00		

The logistic regression model was statistically significant concerning the simulator position parameter, which influences the students' competence level (Table 4). The model's sensitivity was 0% with 100% specificity, the positive predictive value cannot be calculated, and the negative predictive value was 65%. The comparison of the participant's perceptions about the two teaching methodologies showed that procedure-specific videos through E-learning helped the participants in the repetition of skills (4.70 ± 0.398), can be used as an adjunct teaching tool (4.26 ± 0.395), made the participants feel more competent in performing the skill-based procedure (4.30 ± 0.564), and helped the participants to better understand the preclinical practical lab skills (4.20 ± 0.538).

4. Discussion

The dentistry curriculum emphasizes developing psychomotor skills to effectively and judiciously treat patients [18]. The psychomotor skills training for dental undergraduates in operative dentistry starts in the preclinical laboratory. These preclinical laboratories are the foundation stones for inculcating the expertise required to treat patients in clinics during their clinical curriculum. Traditionally, preclinical procedures are taught with the help of live demonstrations in preclinical laboratories [21,22]. This study has found that the students who were given procedure-specific video demonstrations were more competent in preclinical skills than students taught in traditional learning. Khalaf K et al., in their study, concluded that video-assisted learning as an additional tool to traditional teaching could augment the understanding and learning process of students [17]. Thilakumara IP et al. have found in their study that there was a statistically significant difference in terms of improvement of knowledge in the group that used the procedural video [18]. Fayaz A et al., in their study, concluded that instructional videotapes could aid in teaching the fabrication of complete dentures and are as effective as the traditional teaching system [23]. Recently, Elham Soltanimehr has documented that the virtual method of learning was better for acquiring knowledge than the traditional lecture-based learning during the diagnostic imaging of bone lesions of the jaw [20].

The competency level showed no significant difference between the control group and experimental group before the intervention, indicating the same level of knowledge and competency of dental undergraduates participating in the study. After the intervention, the experimental group in which procedure-specific video demonstration was given, has shown a significant difference. Similar results are obtained in other studies [24]. These differences in the competency level before and after the intervention can be contributed by the fact that video demonstrations enable the student to visualize the procedure [18]. At the same time, it might help them recall the process and implement it in preclinical activities [18]. The procedure-specific educational videos are vital because they allow the students visual and mental practice and enhance their psychomotor skills during the procedures and the novel aspects of learning from videos [25]. Moreover, it is beneficial to acquire technical skills and simulation in clinical settings [20,21]. However, contrarily, some studies have found no difference in the competency level of the students, whether they have been given a video demonstration or traditional teaching [26]. Because the students have different psychomotor skill levels, dividing them into other groups and evaluating the effect of the two methods might not necessarily show the real impact [26].

In the preclinical skill of operative dentistry, cavity preparation and restoration are the main procedures. They involve multiple steps, which second-year undergraduate dental students should master. These steps may range from general steps, including infection control, simulator and operator position, and tray organization, to the specific steps of cavity preparation, including cavity outline, resistance form and retention form. Therefore, students' understanding and mastering of these steps were crucial and were evaluated using two different teaching methodologies by two other students in this study. When infection control and operator position were compared, male students were 1.60 times at higher risk of noncompliance than females. Contrarily, male students had shown an 81% higher chance of higher competency when the simulator position was compared to female students. Contrarily, some studies have reported no gender variation related to competency level in preclinical prosthodontics laboratory techniques [18].

Similarly, students with low CGPA scores were 2.51 times at higher risk for not showing competence in infection control procedures, 1.41 times at higher risk for not properly arranging the tray, and 2.51 times at higher risk of using incorrect operator position. On specific cavity design, students with low CGPA were 1.70 times at higher risk of competency than high CGPA scores in the resistance form and retention form of cavity preparation. The effect of CGPA could be related to the confidence level of the students. It has been reported that students with high CGPA scores were able to perform specific dental procedures better than the students with low CGPA scores [27].

There has been a considerable debate on implementing newer teaching strategies over the past years. However, in E-learning, the learner may take a more self-directed learning approach. Nevertheless, self-directed learning is one of the essential adult learning methods that can prepare dental students for a successful lifelong career as a dentist [28]. Regardless, if the system is introduced strategically with proper planning, it may influence the students' quality of learning [29]. The procedural video demonstration method helps students to gain knowledge and visualize the steps.

Furthermore, it is a self-paced method, and students are given a chance to watch and understand the procedure by watching the videos multiple times at their convenience. It helps improve levels of motivation, satisfaction and concentration [30]. While in traditional teaching, the instructor gives a live demonstration in a shorter period, and sometimes, a few technical steps are difficult to visualize from one direction. A student may be allowed to repeat the procedure themselves (experiential learning) after a live demonstration. The demonstrator will then assess the student's work and provide constructive feedback [13]. It allows dental students to plan productively for their next learning experience, thereby enabling progress around the experiential (learning by doing) learning cycle. Besides supporting reflection, this feedback also helps students gain a more in-depth understanding of complex subjects.

Moreover, sometimes, there are variations seen in the live demonstrations of different instructors [2–5]. A simulated dental environment is often used for live demonstrations, which is crucial for dental students' familiarity and community of practice. Even so, E-learning may occur in environments other than the dental environment.

While assessing the participant's perception of the teaching methodologies to compare them at the end of this study, we have found that the procedure-specific videos through Blackboard were considered a better teaching methodology than the live demonstration. Therefore, procedure-specific video demonstration can be an alternative method for live demonstrations on five out of seven statements. The finding agreed with the study done by Alqahtani et al., which showed a high mean response for the procedure-specific video group (experimental group) than the live demonstration group (control group) concerning understanding the different steps, visualization, and clarity of the procedure [3]. In a study by Argon and Zibrowski, the participants preferred procedure-specific videos over the live demonstration, claiming that they were able to visualize better and had the liberty to review the procedure at any time as per their convenience and as many times as required [31]. Although every effort was made to standardize the procedure, individual variations of the lab instructor can affect the live demonstration even then.

Although there is a shred of evidence that procedure-specific video-based teaching and learning are preferred methods by students, certain studies show contrasting findings of the participants' attitudes toward procedure-specific video-based learning. A study by Smith et al. found no difference between the attitude of medical students toward the method of teaching and instruction [32]. A novelty of this study is that results were obtained from a comparative group and a control group via convenient sampling. As a control group, it was chosen because small cohorts of students could share resources and learn together.

Many variables can influence the students' competence level in learning practical skills. Educational videos can only be used as adjunct tools, not as alternative tools for the learning process. E-learning tools' most significant limitation is the lack of demonstrator interaction, whereas, in live demonstrations, the demonstrator can clarify students' questions during the demonstration process. Contrarily, the live demonstration could promote the social learning theory of community of practice (students and faculty members are part of a group who share a common interest and a desire to gain knowledge from and contribute to the community with their variety of experiences) [33,34]. Learning by educational videos does not support the concept of directed self-learning. Furthermore, the abrupt online transition of the learning process during COVID-19 can negatively affect legitimacy and validity. Other factors include a lack of practical skills, low attendance due to heavy internet traffic, and student involvement. Despite the contribution of this study to the literature, there are a few unanswered questions. Since this study was conducted on a single cohort of samples from one speciality of dentistry, it is not easy to generalize its results to other branches of dentistry, such as periodontics or prosthodontics. This study shows the longitudinal impact of educational videos on knowledge and skills retention and how it is transferred into safe clinical practice. Research in the future should investigate students' levels of competency in restoring teeth after watching the supplemental videos in clinical practice sessions.

5. Conclusions

The participants taught by hybrid teaching modality proved to be better and demonstrated a higher level of knowledge and skill competency than those who were not. Therefore, we recommend within the scope of this study that additional procedure-specific educational videos and other resources through E-learning should be a part of the teaching methodology for the preclinical operative dentistry skill course to enhance the students' knowledge and skill competency levels.

Author Contributions: Conceptualization, K.K.G., A.I. and M.O.H.; methodology, O.K., D.S., K.C.S., A.M.A.A. and A.A.E.G.A.; formal analysis, K.K.G., K.C.S., B.A., T.A. and A.M.A.A.; writing—original draft preparation, K.K.G., A.I., B.A., D.S. and K.C.S., writing—review and editing, A.A.E.G.A., M.O.H., A.M.A.A., T.A. and O.K. All authors have read and agreed to the published version of the manuscript.

Funding: This research received no external funding.

Institutional Review Board Statement: The study was conducted in accordance with the Declaration of Helsinki and approved by the local committee for bioethics, Jouf University.

Informed Consent Statement: Informed consent was obtained from all subjects involved in the study.

Data Availability Statement: Data will be made available upon request.

Conflicts of Interest: The authors declare no conflict of interest.

References

1. Sahu, P.K.; Chattu, V.K.; Rewatkar, A.; Sakhamuri, S. Best practices to impart clinical skills during preclinical years of medical curriculum. *J. Educ. Health Promot.* **2019**, *8*, 57–64. [PubMed]
2. Kalaskar, R.R.; Kalaskar, A.R. Effectiveness of 3D video system on the performance of students during preclinical Cavity preparation exercise. *J. Educ. Technol. Health Sci.* **2015**, *2*, 57–61.
3. Alqahtani, N.D.; Al-Jewair, T.; Khalid, A.-M.; Albarakati, S.F.; ALkofide, E.A. Live demonstration versus procedural video: A comparison of two methods for teaching an orthodontic laboratory procedure. *BMC Med. Educ.* **2015**, *15*, 1–4. [CrossRef] [PubMed]
4. Karimi Moonaghi, H.; Derakhshan, A.; Valai, N.; Mortazavi, F. The effectiveness of video-based education on gaining practical learning skills in comparison with demonstrating methods effectiveness among university students. *J. Med. Educ.* **2003**, *4*, 27–30.
5. Buchanan, J.A. Use of simulation technology in dental education. *J. Dent. Educ.* **2001**, *65*, 1225–1231. [CrossRef]
6. Bhola, S.; Hellyer, P. The risks and benefits of social media in dental foundation training. *Br. Dent. J.* **2016**, *221*, 609–613. [CrossRef] [PubMed]
7. Naser-Ud-Din, S. Introducing scenario based learning interactive to postgraduates in UQ Orthodontic Program. *Eur. J. Dent. Educ.* **2015**, *19*, 169–176. [CrossRef]
8. Hillenburg, K.; Cederberg, R.; Gray, S.; Hurst, C.; Johnson, G.; Potter, B. E-learning and the future of dental education: Opinions of administrators and information technology specialists. *Eur. J. Dent. Educ.* **2006**, *10*, 169–177. [CrossRef]
9. Cook, D.A.; Erwin, P.J.; Triola, M.M. Computerized virtual patients in health professions education: A systematic review and meta-analysis. *Acad. Med.* **2010**, *85*, 1589–1602. [CrossRef] [PubMed]
10. Hempel, G.; Neef, M.; Rotzoll, D.; Heinke, W. Study of medicine 2.0 due to Web 2.0?!-risks and opportunities for the curriculum in Leipzig. *GMS Z. Med. Ausbild.* **2013**, *30*, 10–17.
11. Jarczewski, A.; Balzer, F.; Stötzner, P.; Ahlers, O. GMS Journal for Medical Education. *GMS Z. Med. Ausbild.* **2013**, *30*, 1.
12. Mahmoodi, B.; Sagheb, K.; Sagheb, K.; Schulz, P.; Willershausen, B.; Al-Nawas, B.; Walter, C. Catalogue of interactive learning objectives to improve an integrated medical and dental curriculum. *J. Contemp. Dent. Pract.* **2016**, *17*, 965–968. [CrossRef] [PubMed]
13. Modha, B. Experiential learning without prior vicarious learning: An insight from the primary dental care setting. *Educ. Prim. Care* **2021**, *32*, 49–55. [CrossRef] [PubMed]
14. AlKarani, A.S.; Thobaity, A.A. Medical Staff Members' Experiences with Blackboard at Taif University, Saudi Arabia. *J. Multidiscip. Healthc.* **2020**, *13*, 1629. [CrossRef]
15. Ramlogan, S.; Raman, V.; Sweet, J. A comparison of two forms of teaching instruction: Video vs. live lecture for education in clinical periodontology. *Eur. J. Dent. Educ.* **2014**, *18*, 31–38. [CrossRef]
16. Zitzmann, N.U.; Matthisson, L.; Ohla, H.; Joda, T. Digital undergraduate education in dentistry: A systematic review. *Int. J. Environ. Res. Public Health* **2020**, *17*, 3269. [CrossRef] [PubMed]
17. Khalaf, K.; El-Kishawi, M.; Mustafa, S.; Al Kawas, S. Effectiveness of technology-enhanced teaching and assessment methods of undergraduate preclinical dental skills: A systematic review of randomized controlled clinical trials. *BMC Med. Educ.* **2020**, *20*, 1–13. [CrossRef] [PubMed]
18. Thilakumara, I.P.; Jayasinghe, R.M.; Rasnayaka, S.K.; Jayasinghe, V.P.; Abeysundara, S. Effectiveness of procedural video versus live demonstrations in teaching laboratory techniques to dental students. *J. Dent. Educ.* **2018**, *82*, 898–904. [CrossRef]
19. Wong, G.; Apthorpe, H.C.; Ruiz, K.; Nanayakkara, S. An innovative educational approach in using instructional videos to teach dental local anaesthetic skills. *Eur. J. Dent. Educ.* **2019**, *23*, 28–34. [CrossRef] [PubMed]
20. Soltanimehr, E.; Bahrampour, E.; Imani, M.M.; Rahimi, F.; Almasi, B.; Moattari, M. Effect of virtual versus traditional education on theoretical knowledge and reporting skills of dental students in radiographic interpretation of bony lesions of the jaw. *BMC Med. Educ.* **2019**, *19*, 1–7. [CrossRef] [PubMed]
21. Botelho, M.; Gao, X.; Jagannathan, N. A qualitative analysis of students' perceptions of videos to support learning in a psychomotor skills course. *Eur. J. Dent. Educ.* **2019**, *23*, 20–27. [PubMed]
22. Asghar, S. Impact of Procedure Specific Videos in the Performance of Restorative Procedures by Pre-Clinical dentistry Students. *JPDA* **2019**, *28*, 176–180.
23. Fayaz, A.; Mazahery, A.; Hosseinzadeh, M.; Yazdanpanah, S. Video-based learning versus traditional method for preclinical course of complete denture fabrication. *J. Dent.* **2015**, *16*, 21.
24. Jeyapalan, K.; Mani, U.M.; Christian, J.; Seenivasan, M.K.; Natarajan, P.; Vaidhyanathan, A.K. Influence of Teaching Strategies and its Order of Exposure on Pre-Clinical Teeth Arrangement—A Pilot Study. *J. Clin. Diagn. Res. JCDR* **2016**, *10*, ZC93. [CrossRef] [PubMed]
25. Naseri, M.; Shantiaee, Y.; Rasekhi, J.; Zadsirjan, S.; Bidabadi, M.M.; Khayat, A. Efficacy of video-assisted instruction on knowledge and performance of dental students in access cavity preparation. *Iran. Endod. J.* **2016**, *11*, 329. [PubMed]
26. Almohareb, T. A comparison between video and live demonstrations for teaching dental operative procedures. *Pak. Oral Dent. J.* **2016**, *36*, 619–622.
27. Baidas, L. Comparison of the Con idence Level of Final Year Dental Students in General Practice between two Saudi Dental Colleges in Riyadh". *EC Dent. Sci.* **2017**, *8*, 38–47.
28. Sandars, J.; Walsh, K. Self-directed learning. *Educ. Prim. Care* **2016**, *27*, 151–152. [CrossRef] [PubMed]

29. Gopinath, V.; Nallaswamy, D. A systematic review on the most effective method teaching dentistry to dental students compared to video based learning. *Am. J. Educ. Res.* **2017**, *5*, 63–68.
30. Garbin, C.A.S.; Pacheco Filho, A.C.; Garbin, A.J.I.; Pacheco, K.T.D.S. Instructional video as a teaching/learning tool in times of remote education: A viable alternative. *J. Dent. Educ.* **2021**, *85*, 2034–2035. [CrossRef] [PubMed]
31. Aragon, C.E.; Zibrowski, E.M. Does exposure to a procedural video enhance preclinical dental student performance in fixed prosthodontics? *J. Dent. Educ.* **2008**, *72*, 67–71. [CrossRef] [PubMed]
32. Smith, A.R.; Cavanaugh, C.; Moore, W.A. Instructional multimedia: An investigation of student and instructor attitudes and student study behavior. *BMC Med. Educ.* **2011**, *11*, 1–13. [CrossRef]
33. Abidi, S.S.R. Healthcare knowledge sharing: Purpose, practices, and prospects. In *Healthcare Knowledge Management*; Springer: Berlin/Heidelberg, Germany, 2007; pp. 67–86.
34. Khattak, O.; Ganji, K.K.; Iqbal, A.; Alonazi, M.; Algarni, H.; Alsharari, T. Educational Videos as an Adjunct Learning Tool in Pre-Clinical Operative Dentistry—A Randomized Control Trial. *Healthcare* **2022**, *10*, 178. [CrossRef]

International Journal of
Environmental Research and Public Health

MDPI

Article

Comparison of Interactive Teaching in Online and Offline Platforms among Dental Undergraduates

Deepak Nallaswamy Veeraiyan [1], Sheeja S. Varghese [2,*], Arvina Rajasekar [2], Mohmed Isaqali Karobari [3,4,*], Lakshmi Thangavelu [5], Anand Marya [6], Pietro Messina [7] and Giuseppe Alessandro Scardina [7,*]

1 Department of Prosthodontics, Saveetha Dental College and Hospitals, Saveetha Institute of Medical and Technical Sciences, Chennai 600077, India; drdeepaknallu@gmail.com
2 Department of Periodontology, Saveetha Dental College and Hospitals, Saveetha Institute of Medical and Technical Sciences, Chennai 600077, India; arvinar.sdc@saveetha.com
3 Department of Conservative Dentistry & Endodontics, Saveetha Dental College and Hospitals, Saveetha Institute of Medical and Technical Sciences, Chennai 600077, India
4 Conservative Dentistry Unit, School of Dental Sciences, Universiti Sains Malaysia, Kota Bharu 16150, Malaysia
5 Department of Pharmacology, Saveetha Dental College and Hospital, Saveetha Institute of Medical and Technical Sciences, Saveetha University, Chennai 600077, India; Lakshmi@saveetha.com
6 Department of Orthodontics, Faculty of Dentistry, University of Puthisastra, Phnom Penh 12211, Cambodia; amarya@puthisastra.edu.kh
7 Department of Surgical, Oncological and Stomatological Disciplines, University of Palermo, 90133 Palermo, Italy; pietro.messina01@unipa.it
* Correspondence: sheeja@saveetha.com (S.S.V.); dr.isaq@gmail.com (M.I.K.); alessandro.scardina@unipa.it (G.A.S.)

Citation: Veeraiyan, D.N.; Varghese, S.S.; Rajasekar, A.; Karobari, M.I.; Thangavelu, L.; Marya, A.; Messina, P.; Scardina, G.A. Comparison of Interactive Teaching in Online and Offline Platforms among Dental Undergraduates. *Int. J. Environ. Res. Public Health* **2022**, *19*, 3170. https://doi.org/10.3390/ijerph19063170

Academic Editors: Paul B. Tchounwou and Kelvin Afrashtehfar

Received: 20 January 2022
Accepted: 4 March 2022
Published: 8 March 2022

Abstract: In recent years, the educational system has focused more on the holistic development of an individual. Modern technology has changed the educational environment to provide students with better academic opportunities. Along with the education system, teaching techniques and learning tools have also changed with digital evolution. This research was undertaken to assess the academic performance of interactive teaching methods in offline and online platforms in Periodontics among BDS undergraduates at a dental college in India. This prospective study was conducted among 49 students: Group I (n = 24, online class through Zoom) and Group II (n = 25, offline classes). The subject was divided into three modules and was covered in one week. The topics covered, teaching methods, lectures, and activities were similar for both groups. A formative assessment mark was obtained from written tests during the module, whereas the summative assessment mark was recorded from exams conducted towards the end of the module. In the results, a statistically significant difference was not observed in terms of formative assessment between Group I (77.88 ± 12.89) and Group II (77.80 ± 16.09) (p = 0.98). In addition, a statistically significant difference was not observed in terms of summative assessment between Group I (80.54 ± 8.39) and Group II (80.28 ± 11.57) (p = 0.93). Overall, this study suggests that interactive teaching methods in both offline and online platforms in Periodontics showed equivalent performance by the undergraduate dental students.

Keywords: dentistry; digital education; education; e-learning; interactive teaching; online teaching

1. Introduction

The education system has evolved dramatically over the years. Classroom-based education systems existed for many years until the modern education system came into the picture in the nineteenth century. The fundamental strength of this modern education system is a well-defined and structured curriculum that gives importance to all the subjects. However, it does not focus on the holistic development of an individual. In addition, it is not easy to create a customized study plan to meet the needs of each individual [1].

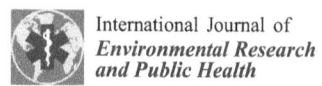

Along with the education system, teaching techniques and learning tools have also changed with digital evolution. Small group learning, rather than traditional lecture-based

learning, is incorporated into the current educational system, which is student-centered. This learning method helps the students express and communicate their thoughts with their peers [2]. In addition, to gain the students' attention, topics are broken down into microlectures and are coupled with activities such as mind mapping, critical pedagogy, and role play. This keeps students engaged and active throughout the session. This didactic and non-didactic method promotes learning and the application of concepts, as well. The primary tactic of this interactive model of learning method should be to exemplify the performance of every student and inculcate exploratory and innovative thinking with flexible training programs in which students can learn at their own pace [3].

An interactive teaching style is a learning activity in which students participate in the process of learning and reflect on what they know, think, and believe. Against conventional methods of teaching, which place a premium on the instructors' prominent role in assisting and facilitating students, the interactive mode of teaching places a premium on the students' abilities and interests [4]. In the conventional classroom method, the instructor is the focus in the learning process, and students are just recipients, but in a student-centered system, the instructor and the student exchange roles, allowing the student to participate diligently in the process of learning, and they become the main focus. The main aim of the instructor or tutor in an interactive mode of learning is to help students achieve their goals. Here, the instructor creates a plan that includes activities, discussions, and problem-solving tasks that allow students to acquire new ideas and change an individual into a group task. Each person in the group contributes to the overall success of the group. The essential components of interactive lessons are interactive activities and tasks that students achieve. Therefore, this method ensures the complete involvement of students throughout learning [5]. The assignments provided in the interactive sessions also help the participants gain knowledge and make them competent enough to complete it with innovative ideas. In addition, the interactive mode of teaching ensures that every participant is actively engaged in intellectual development and everyone offers and shares their opinions, ideas, and information [6].

Furthermore, this allows students to develop multiple skills, such as listening to others, teamwork, analyzing diverse points of view, discussing, and decision making. According to the literature, interactive learning aids the student in acquiring information and retaining it for a prolonged period. It also activates students' creative thinking and analytic and syllogistic skills, allowing them to make reasonable decisions in any situation in order to develop the most acceptable models of thinking, action, and communication [7].

E-learning is becoming more popular in many higher education institutions recently. Both learners and educators are drawn to the benefits of e-learning, which include the ability to learn anywhere, at any time, and at one's own pace. E-learning is distributing educational information to students who are separated by a significant distance from their instructors or teachers. It makes use of the Internet, computers, networks, and multimedia technology [8]. When it comes to e-learning, it is common to use different methods. Learning through this mode can hold the students' attention because it frequently includes interactive images, texts, audio, videos, collaborative sharing, and other features. This also permits interactive learning. Furthermore, we may access information from anywhere and anytime as long as we have a computer and an internet connection. E-learning has the potential to improve educational and training access and teaching and learning quality. It also emphasizes the importance of higher education institutions maintaining a competitive edge in this constantly shifting student market. In addition, here, technology has been fully utilized in improving the teaching and learning process while also allowing for the delivery of educational programs to a more significant number of students at a lower cost. As a result, e-learning can enhance the quality of teaching and learning [9].

The progress of society and the impact of technology are directly related to the quality of education. Different students respond to various instructional methods. Some people learn better by seeing things, while others prefer reading or listening to lectures. To combat this, teachers provide students with various possibilities and routes to comprehend better topics, such as videos and other digital web resources in place of traditional learning content. The online platform has gained importance recently due to the COVID-19 pandemic. This panic and the accessibility to internet facilities lead to various online education programs on platforms such as Zoom or Google Classroom. Progressive learning on such platforms allows students to move away from their workstations and learn independently. Students can study actively and participate in experimental learning with this freedom [10].

Implementing interactive teaching methods in periodontics enhances students' critical thinking skills and improves their curiosity and logical reasoning in simplifying complex subject matters [11]. Furthermore, interactive education increases interaction and permits users to participate in the information, making it a more active, student-centered model. Another retrospective study among postgraduate dental students suggested that interactive teaching methods considerably improved the students' academic performance [12]. Similarly, active learning strategies have been demonstrated to promote learning and understanding in subjects such as preclinical endodontics, forensic odontology, and pathology [13–15].

In addition, learning through e-classes was equally effective compared to conventional classroom teachings among medical students [16,17]. A cross-sectional study assessed the utility of online teaching among dental students, and it was found that the majority of the students liked online teaching [18]. However, the comparison of academic performance of interactive teaching methods in offline and online platforms in undergraduate dental programs has not been studied. This research was undertaken to assess whether there is any difference in academic performance of interactive teaching methods in offline and online platforms in Periodontics among undergraduate dental students at a dental college in India.

2. Materials and Methods

This study was approved by the Institutional Review Board of Saveetha Dental College and Hospitals, Tamil Nadu, India. This prospective study was conducted at Saveetha Dental College and Hospitals, Tamil Nadu, India, where the subject Periodontics was taught in interactive teaching method in an offline and online platform for undergraduates of the final year based on Bachelor of Dental Surgery curriculum.

The current study enrolled a total of 56 students. The students were given the option to choose either an online or offline class. Among 56 students, 27 students opted for an online class through Zoom (Group I), and 29 students opted for an offline class (Group II). The teaching plan was created for 1 week. The subject was divided into three modules: Module 1—Introduction and Etiopathogenesis of periodontal disease; Module 2—Diseases of the periodontium; and Module 3—Diagnosis and Treatment. Each module was further subdivided into 12 lectures.

Module 1 was discussed under introduction, gingiva, periodontal ligament, cementum, alveolar bone, age changes of the periodontium, dental plaque and calculus, influence of systemic diseases on the periodontium, environmental and genetic factors, iatrogenic factors, microbiology, and immunology. Module 2 was divided into the classification of gingival diseases, classification of periodontal diseases, stages of gingival inflammation, clinical features of gingivitis, gingival enlargement, acute gingival lesions, abscesses of the periodontium, periodontal pocket, periodontitis, necrotizing ulcerative conditions, patterns of bone loss, and the role of occlusion in periodontal disease. Module 3 was taught under the following headings: risk factors, prognosis, conventional diagnostic methods, advanced diagnostic methods, instruments and instrumentation, non-surgical periodontal therapy, gingival surgical procedures, periodontal flap surgery, regenerative periodontal therapy, resective periodontal therapy, furcation involvement and management, and mucogingival surgeries.

An interactive method of teaching was used for each module. Offline teaching consisted of lectures on specific topics, which lasted 20 min. Each lecture was followed by in-class activities such as concept mapping, quizzes, role playing, puzzle, and crosswords which lasted for 20 to 40 min. The online class was conducted via Zoom classroom, and it also consisted of lectures followed by activities. In order to avoid bias, similar activities were given to the students who opted for an online platform. It was made sure that the same interactive teaching method was conducted online for Group I students. All 3 modules were completed in 36 h for both groups. The topics covered, teaching methods, lectures, and activities were identical for both sets of students.

During each module, written tests were conducted for both the groups and were scored separately and added together to obtain a cumulative formative assessment. The students in groups I and II were given a summative score based on their performance on the written exam at the end of the module. (Figure 1). All the exam time limits were constant for both groups. In addition, the exams were monitored throughout the session.

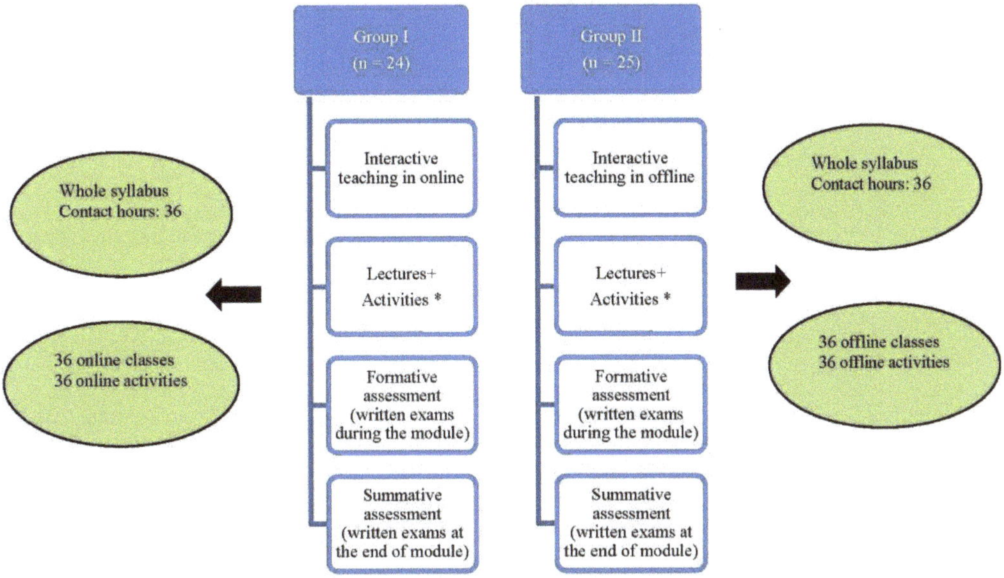

Figure 1. Schematic representation of interactive teaching in the online and offline platform. * 20 min lecture and 20–40 min activity from 8 a.m.–3 p.m. for 1 week.

The same examiner carried out both summative and formative assessments for groups I and II. In addition, the university's third-year marks were obtained to avoid bias about the academic prospects of the two groups. The Kolmogorov–Smirnov test and the Shapiro–Wilk test of normality were used to evaluate the results. The results followed a parametric distribution according to the data. An unpaired *t*-test was used to compare the two groups' scores on the summative and formative exams. Statistical Package for Social Sciences (SPSS Software, Version 23.0; IBM Corp., Armonk, NY, USA) was used to analyze the data. When the *p*-value was <0.05, the results were considered statistically significant.

3. Results

In the present study, 27 students opted for an online class through Zoom (Group I), and 29 students opted for offline class (Group II). Three students from Group I and four students from Group II failed to attend any of the modules or exams conducted during the module. Those students were excluded from the final data analysis. For statistical analysis, 24 students from Group I and 25 students from Group II were considered (Figure 2).

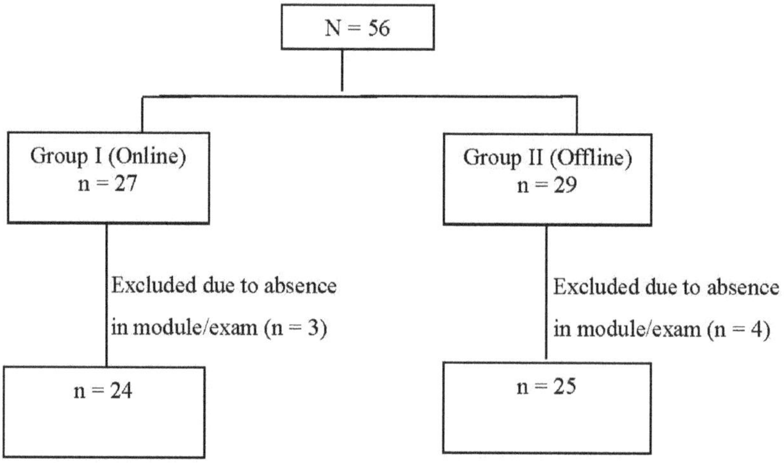

Figure 2. Study flow chart.

Students in both groups were compared based on formative and summative assessments. The unpaired *t*-test revealed no significant difference between the students' academic performance in both groups during their third year (p = 0.423). (Table 1)

Table 1. Comparison of third-year examination marks between the two groups.

Variables	Groups	Mean ± SD	*t*-Value	*p*-Value
Examination marks	Group I Group II	74.25 ± 10.71 76.64 ± 10.003	−0.808	0.423

The independent *t*-test was used to compare both groups' formative assessment scores during the module. We discovered no significant difference (p = 0.98) between groups. The summative evaluation scores of both groups were compared using an independent *t*-test. No difference (p = 0.93) between groups were observed. (Table 2)

Table 2. Comparison of formative and summative assessment marks between the two groups.

Variables	Groups	Mean ± SD	*t*-Value	*p*-Value
Formative assessment marks	Group I Group II	77.88 ± 12.89 77.80 ± 16.09	0.018	0.98
Summative assessment marks	Group I Group II	80.54 ± 8.39 80.28 ± 11.57	0.090	0.93

4. Discussion

The present study assessed the academic performance of interactive teaching methods in offline and online platforms in Periodontics among undergraduate dental students. For both groups of students, didactic and non-didactic teaching methods were implemented. The same teaching method was conducted online for the Group I students and in the classroom for the Group II students. According to the results, the performance was similar between the two groups in terms of formative and summative evaluation marks.

Several studies have demonstrated that interactive teaching mode was as excellent as conventional teaching methods, and in certain trials, it was proven to be the most effective learning approach [13–22]. Compared to traditional teaching approaches, interactive teaching has a considerable impact on cognitive achievement and learning attitude. In addition, for a wide range of learning outcomes, interactive teaching approaches have repeatedly been demonstrated to be equally as effective and, in some cases, more effective than traditional methods. A study by Veeraiyan DN et al. introduced the Multiple Interactive Learning Algorithm (MILA) in teaching Periodontics among undergraduate dental students. The study revealed that implementing interactive teaching methods that include a lecture followed by a game-based learning activity enhances the students' performance [11]. In another study, video-based learning was implemented for one group of students, and another group of students received video-based lectures along with in-class activities. It was suggested that the blended module-based teaching resulted in significant improvement in the in-course assessments [13]. Our results are similar as the students in both groups showed improved performance in examinations, suggesting that the interactive teaching method was effective irrespective of the mode of teaching.

When students' progress was compared with and without using technology throughout teaching, no difference was found between the classroom and distance learning groups [16]. Singh K et al. assessed the merits and demerits of online classes among dental students [17]. Most participants reported that they were allowed to interact and clarify their doubts with the teacher than they experienced in the actual classroom. In addition, an equal number of students thought both the actual classroom and the e-classroom were effective. The responses were also consistent across semesters. In addition, there was no significant difference in average marks between the two groups when structured interactive lectures were compared to traditional lectures as a teaching approach for pharmacology. However, a questionnaire analysis of the students' perceptions revealed that they preferred the structured interactive teaching technique. Furthermore, interactive approaches and strategies such as flipped classrooms and multiple-choice questions in interactive mode engage students in the learning process, allowing them to retain more information and hence feel pleased [18].

Bains M et al., in their study, assessed the acceptance of didactic and non-didactic interactive methods of learning in the classroom and in online platforms among dental undergraduates in learning cephalometric tracing in Orthodontics. The findings revealed that students favored interactive teaching methods, implying that both online and offline sessions were practical and well-received [23]. This is in accordance with the present study, as the interactive mode of teaching improved the academic performance of the students in both the groups. In addition, Ochoa JG et al. suggested that an interactive style incorporating Web technology improves seizure disorder learning, maybe by stimulating critical thinking and increasing student motivation [24]. Similar results were obtained when the effectiveness of interactive teaching using media was assessed for teaching interpretation of arterial blood gas to medical students was compared to traditional lecture-based models [25]. Our findings are in agreement with the previous studies. In addition, our study finding highlights that interactive teaching method in both offline and online platforms resulted in significant growth in competence on the topics covered in all the three modules.

In addition, studies have demonstrated that e-learning may promote learning comparable to classroom lectures [26,27]. Another cross-sectional study evaluated the merits of e-learning among medical postgraduates after one month of online teaching, and it was suggested that e-learning is a viable alternative to classroom learning [28]. Similarly, studies by Bischoff W R et al. [29] and Gragan M K et al. [30] reported that there was no difference between traditional classroom learning and e-learning in terms of performance. Overall, our findings follow that of other studies.

The student's intellectual ability might be a confounding factor; however, there was no significant difference between the two students' third-year marks. In addition, the question paper used during the module and at the end of the module may not be a confounding factor because the questions were carefully designed for both sets of students to be of the same difficulty level.

The study design may be a potential limitation of the research. The study is not a randomized trial because students were given the option of learning in one of two platforms. Other flaws include the small sample size and a single study center, restricting the generalizability of the findings. More randomized clinical studies in a broader context are needed to obtain more data on the efficacy of various teaching methods.

5. Conclusions

This study found that interactive teaching methods in both offline and online platforms in Periodontics resulted in equivalent performance by the undergraduate dental students. Both the groups were benefited equally by interacting teaching method. Therefore, interactive teaching methods, either offline or online, provide students a beneficial learning environment.

Author Contributions: Conceptualization, D.N.V., S.S.V. and M.I.K.; methodology, A.R. and L.T.; software, M.I.K.; validation, A.M., P.M. and G.A.S.; formal analysis, D.N.V.; investigation, S.S.V.; resources, L.T. and A.R.; data curation, A.R., and L.T.; writing—original draft preparation, S.S.V., A.R. and A.M.; writing—review and editing, P.M. and G.A.S.; visualization, D.N.V.; supervision, S.S.V., M.I.K. and G.A.S.; project administration, D.N.V. and S.S.V.; funding acquisition, P.M. and G.A.S. All authors have read and agreed to the published version of the manuscript.

Funding: This research received no external funding.

Institutional Review Board Statement: The study was conducted according to the guidelines of the Declaration of Helsinki and approved by the Institutional Human Ethical Committee of Saveetha dental college and hospitals (IHEC/SDC/FACULTY/21/PERIO/302).

Informed Consent Statement: Informed consent was obtained from all subjects involved in the study.

Data Availability Statement: Any data related to the study can be provided by the authors on reasonable request.

Conflicts of Interest: The authors declare no conflict of interest.

References

1. Hargreaves, A.; Goodson, I. Educational change over time? The sustainability and non sustainability of three decades of secondary school change and continuity. *Educ. Adm. Q.* **2006**, *42*, 3–41. [CrossRef]
2. Hommes, J.; Arah, O.A.; de Grave, W.; Schuwirth, L.W.; Scherpbier, A.J.; Bos, G.M. Medical students perceive better group learning processes when large classes are made to seem small. *PLoS ONE* **2014**, *9*, e93328. [CrossRef] [PubMed]
3. Hanson, D. *Instructor's Guide to Process-Oriented Guided-Inquiry Learning*; Pacific Crest: Lisle, IL, USA, 2006.
4. Burgess, A.; Bleasel, J.; Haq, I.; Roberts, C.; Garsia, R.; Robertson, T.; Mellis, C. Team-based learning (TBL) in the medical curriculum: Better than PBL. *BMC Med. Educ.* **2017**, *17*, 243. [CrossRef] [PubMed]
5. Freeman, S.; Eddy, S.L.; McDonough, M.; Smith, M.K.; Okoroafor, N.; Jordt, H.; Wenderoth, M.P. Active learning increases student performance in science, engineering, and mathematics. *Proc. Natl. Acad. Sci. USA* **2014**, *111*, 8410–8415. [CrossRef] [PubMed]
6. Black, E.W.; Blue, A.V.; Davidson, R.; McCormack, W.T. Using team-based learning in a large interprofessional health science education experience. *J. Interprof. Educ. Pract.* **2016**, *5*, 19–22. [CrossRef]
7. Kleffner, J.H.; Dadian, T. Using collaborative learning in dental education. *J. Dent. Educ.* **1997**, *61*, 66–72. [CrossRef]
8. Gond, R.; Gupt, R. A study on digital education in India: Scope and challenges of an indian society. *Anveshana's Int. J. Res. Reg. Stud. Law Soc. Sci. J. Manag. Pract.* **2017**, *2*, 12–18.
9. Hurlbut, A.R. Online vs. traditional learning in teacher education: A comparison of student progress. *Am. J. Distance Educ.* **2018**, *32*, 248–266. [CrossRef]
10. Tokareva, E.A.; Smirnova, Y.V.; Orchakova, L.G. Innovation and communication technologies: Analysis of the effectiveness of their use and implementation in higher education. *Educ. Inf. Technol.* **2019**, *24*, 3219–3234. [CrossRef]
11. Sheeja Varghese, D.R.; Maliappan, S.; Ramamurthy, J.; Murugan, T.; Lochana, P.; Gajendran, D.R. MILA in teaching Periodontics. *Int. J. Pharm. Res.* **2020**, *12*, 2755–2767. [CrossRef]
12. Varghese, S.S.; Ramesh, A.; Veeraiyan, D.N. Blended Module-Based Teaching in Biostatistics and Research Methodology: A Retrospective Study with Postgraduate Dental Students. *J. Dent. Educ.* **2019**, *83*, 445–450. [CrossRef] [PubMed]
13. Veeraiyan, D.N.; Sekhar, P. Critical appraisal-based learning in a dental college in India: A randomized control study. *J. Dent. Educ.* **2013**, *77*, 1079–1085. [CrossRef] [PubMed]
14. Manuel, M.L. Comparative Study Between Conventional and Module Based Forensic Odontology Classes; A Questionnaire Based Cross-Sectional Study among Students of Saveetha Dental College. *Int. J. Res. Trends Innov.* **2021**, *6*, 130–134.
15. Prashaanthi, N.; Brundha, M.P. A Comparative Study between Popplet Notes and Conventional Notes for Learning Pathology. *Res. J. Pharm. Technol.* **2018**, *11*, 175–178. [CrossRef]

16. Jaber, M.; Al-Samarrai, B.; Al-Obaidee, A.; Varma, S.R.; Karobari, M.I.; Marya, A. Does general and specific traits of personality predict students' academic performance? *Biomed Res. Int.* **2022**, *2022*, 1–8. [CrossRef] [PubMed]
17. Singh, K.; Srivastav, S.; Bhardwaj, A.; Dixit, A.; Misra, S. Medical education during the COVID-19 pandemic: A single institution experience. *Indian Pediatr.* **2020**, *57*, 678–679. [CrossRef] [PubMed]
18. Chilwant, K.S. Comparison of two teaching methods, structured interactive lectures and conventional lectures. *Biomed. Res.* **2012**, *23*, 363–366.
19. Afrashtehfar, K.I.; Bryant, S.R. Understanding the lived experience of North American dental patients with a single-tooth implant in the upper front region of the mouth: Protocol for a qualitative study. *JMIR Res. Protoc.* **2021**, *10*, e25767. [CrossRef]
20. Afrashtehfar, K.I. Comments about the appraisal of systematic reviews in restorative dentistry. *F1000Research* **2021**, *10*, 442. [CrossRef]
21. Afrashtehfar, K.I.; Eimar, H.; Yassine, R.; Abi-Nader, S.; Tamimi, F. Evidence-based dentistry for planning restorative treatments: Barriers and potential solutions. *Eur. J. Dent. Educ.* **2017**, *21*, e7–e18. [CrossRef]
22. Luke, A.M.; Mathew, S.; Kuriadom, S.T.; George, J.M.; Karobari, M.I.; Marya, A.; Pawar, A.M. Effectiveness of problem-based learning versus traditional teaching methods in improving acquisition of radiographic interpretation skills among dental students—a systematic review and meta-analysis. *Biomed Res. Int.* **2021**. [CrossRef] [PubMed]
23. Bains, M.; Reynolds, P.A.; McDonald, F.; Sherriff, M. Effectiveness and acceptability of face-to-face, blended and e-learning: A randomized trial of orthodontic undergraduates. *Eur. J. Dent. Educ.* **2011**, *15*, 110–117. [CrossRef] [PubMed]
24. Ochoa, J.G.; Wludyka, P. Randomized comparison between traditional and traditional plus interactive Web-based methods for teaching seizure disorders. *Teach. Learn. Med.* **2008**, *20*, 114–117. [CrossRef]
25. Armstrong, P.; Elliott, T.; Ronald, J.; Paterson, B. Comparison of traditional and interactive teaching methods in a UK emergency department. *Eur. J. Emerg. Med.* **2009**, *16*, 327–329. [CrossRef]
26. Srivastava, V.; Pandey, V.; Tiwari, P.; Patel, S.; Ansari, M.A.; Shukla, V.K. Utility of real-time online teaching during COVID era among surgery postgraduates. *Indian J. Surg.* **2020**, *82*, 762–768. [CrossRef] [PubMed]
27. Huynh, R. The role of E-learning in medical education. *Acad. Med.* **2017**, *92*, 430. [CrossRef]
28. Pather, N.; Blyth, P.; Chapman, J.A.; Dayal, M.R.; Flack, N.A.; Fogg, Q.A.; Green, R.A.; Hulme, A.K.; Johnson, I.P.; Meyer, A.J.; et al. Forced disruption of anatomy education in Australia and New Zealand: An acute response to the COVID-19 pandemic. *Anat. Sci. Educ.* **2020**, *13*, 284–300. [CrossRef]
29. Bischoff, W.R. Transactional Distance, Interactive Television, and Electronic Mail Communication in Graduate Public Health and Nursing Courses: Implications for Professional Education. Ph.D. Thesis, University of Hawai'i at Manoa, Honolulu, HI, USA, 1993.
30. Gragan, M.K. Comparison of learning outcomes between graduates students in telecourses and those in traditional classrooms. Keck JF. J Nurs Educ 31: 229–234, 1992. *J. Phys. Ther. Educ.* **1994**, *8*, 80–81. [CrossRef]

International Journal of
Environmental Research and Public Health

MDPI

Article

Knowledge of COVID-19 Infection Guidelines among the Dental Health Care Professionals of Jazan Region, Saudi Arabia

Syed Nahid Basheer [1,*], Thilla Sekar Vinothkumar [1], Nassreen Hassan Mohammad Albar [1], Mohmed Isaqali Karobari [2,3,4,*], Apathsakayan Renugalakshmi [5], Ahmed Bokhari [5], Syed Wali Peeran [6], Syed Ali Peeran [6], Loai Mohammed Alhadri [7] and Santosh Kumar Tadakamadla [8]

1 Department of Restorative Dental Sciences, College of Dentistry, Jazan University, Jazan 45142, Saudi Arabia; vsekar@jazanu.edu.sa (T.S.V.); nalbar@jazanu.edu.sa (N.H.M.A.)
2 Conservative Dentistry Unit, School of Dental Sciences, Universiti Sains Malaysia, Health Campus, Kubang Kerian, Kota Bharu 16150, Malaysia
3 Center for Transdisciplinary Research (CFTR), Saveetha Dental College & Hospitals, Saveetha Institute of Medical and Technical Sciences University, Chennai 600077, India
4 Department of Restorative Dentistry & Endodontics, Faculty of Dentistry, University of Puthisastra, Phnom Penh 12211, Cambodia
5 Department of Preventive Dental Sciences, College of Dentistry, Jazan University, Jazan 45142, Saudi Arabia; rsakayan@jazanu.edu.sa (A.R.); abokhari@jazanu.edu.sa (A.B.)
6 Department of Periodontics, Armed Forces Hospital, Jazan 82722, Saudi Arabia; doctorsyedwali@yahoo.in (S.W.P.); alipeeran@gmail.com (S.A.P.)
7 Interns Affairs Unit, College of Dentistry, Jazan University, Jazan 45142, Saudi Arabia; 201310090@stu.jazanu.edu.sa
8 School of Medicine and Dentistry, Menzies Health Institute Queensland, Griffith University, Southport, QLD 4222, Australia; santoshkumar.tadakamadla@griffithuni.edu.au
* Correspondence: snbasheer@jazanu.edu.sa (S.N.B.); dr.isaq@gmail.com (M.I.K.)

Abstract: Background: This study aimed to assess the knowledge about guidelines related to COVID-19 infection control procedures among dental health care professionals (DHCPs) in the Jazan region. Methods: A cross-sectional study involving DHCPs (dental students, interns, and dentists) of the Jazan region between January and March 2021. A questionnaire with 35 items was developed and circulated online among the DHCPs. The dimensionality of the questionnaire was assessed using exploratory factor analysis (EFA). The level of awareness (LOA) was compared across the genders, level of professional experience, and exposure to guidelines. Participants were considered to have high LOA when they responded to 26 or more items correctly. Results: A total of 363 DHCPs participated in the survey. The questionnaire was found to be valid and reliable. EFA revealed a distinct three-factor structure. Moreover, 61.2% of the respondents had high LOA related to COVID-19 infection prevention. Among those who had high LOA, dentists (65.5%) were relatively more than the students (62.5%) and interns (46.2%). Among the six guideline statements related explicitly to operative dentistry, more than 50% of the respondents were aware of 3 guideline statements, while less than 50% of the respondents were aware of the remaining statements. Conclusions: Most DHCP had a high LOA for general COVID-19 infection prevention and control guidelines. Dentists, males, and those who read the guidelines had higher LOA than their counterparts.

Keywords: attitude; COVID-19; guidelines; dentistry; operative; infection control; Jazan

Citation: Basheer, S.N.; Vinothkumar, T.S.; Albar, N.H.M.; Karobari, M.I.; Renugalakshmi, A.; Bokhari, A.; Peeran, S.W.; Peeran, S.A.; Alhadri, L.M.; Tadakamadla, S.K. Knowledge of COVID-19 Infection Guidelines among the Dental Health Care Professionals of Jazan Region, Saudi Arabia. *Int. J. Environ. Res. Public Health* **2022**, *19*, 2034. https://doi.org/10.3390/ijerph19042034

Academic Editors: Stefano Pagano and Paul B. Tchounwou

Received: 20 December 2021
Accepted: 8 February 2022
Published: 11 February 2022

1. Introduction

Coronavirus disease 2019 (COVID-19) is caused by the severe acute respiratory syndrome coronavirus 2 (SARS-CoV-2) virus, that spreads from one infected person to another. The virus can spread through the mouth, nose, or eyes in the form of droplets, aerosols, and also sometimes through contaminated surfaces [1,2]. The WHO announced COVID-19 disease as a pandemic on 11th March 2020. According to the World Health Organization [3], as of 1 October 2021, there have been 233,503,524 confirmed cases of COVID-19 globally, including 4,777,503 deaths. As of 2 October 2021, a total of 6,187,643,539 vaccine doses against COVID-19 have been administered [4]. In Saudi Arabia, the first case was reported on 2 March 2020, followed by the lockdown. Subsequently, the dental clinic reopening guidelines were released in June 2020 and updated from time to time [5].

The spread of infection in a dental office occurs either directly through droplets/aerosols or indirectly by contact with mucous membranes, saliva, respiratory fluids, and contaminated surfaces. Most dental procedures generate aerosols, especially in operative dentistry [6]. Aerosol-generating procedures (AGP) have a high potential to transmit the COVID-19 disease [7,8]. Therefore, dental health care providers (DHCP) are at high risk of exposure to SARS-CoV-2, thereby rendering them vulnerable to infection [9,10]. Although the knowledge of DHCP on COVID-19 was acceptable in the previous studies [11,12], it is imperative to ensure that all DHCP have adequate knowledge of the guidelines and their updates to protect patients and the dental team from cross-infection.

Several guidelines for COVID-19 prevention have been published by the Saudi Ministry of Health (MOH), WHO, American Dental Association, Centres for Disease Control and Prevention, and National Health Services to be adopted during the COVID-19 pandemic, which includes maintaining physical distancing, use of well-fitted masks, maintaining adequate ventilation, avoiding crowded indoor spaces, practising good hand hygiene, keeping the environment clean, covering coughs and sneezes with a bent elbow, and getting vaccinated [2,4,5,13,14]. Moreover, various schemes are recommended to reduce the spread of the virus while performing aerosol-generating procedures in a dental setting such as the nonuse of 3 in 1 syringes, the use of high-volume suction, practising four-handed dentistry, and adopting noninvasive procedures such as atraumatic restorative technique [2,5,13,15–17].

It is crucial for all the stakeholders to be aware of the latest guidelines and strictly implement them to mitigate the COVID-19 transmission within the dental care settings [2,4,5,13,14]. As far as the DHCP is concerned, awareness about the general guidelines and operative dentistry needs to be assessed to ensure effective implementation. Operative dentistry is vital for general dental practice because restoring the carious tooth is considered the most common treatment [18]. Awareness about all the necessary protocols, from preparing dental clinics before patient arrival until the patient leaves the dental clinic, must be thoroughly surveyed.

Recently, the DHCP belonging to university dental clinics representing four different regions (Riyadh, Jeddah, Asir and Jazan) of Saudi Arabia have been surveyed for their knowledge on COVID-19. However, the response rate was low, limiting the generalisability of their findings. The authors highlighted the positive impact of timely disseminating national guidelines to all the DHCP on their knowledge [12]. However, the awareness of DHCP about the guideline's statements related to infection prevention and control of COVID-19 in general and during operative procedures, in particular, has not been evaluated.

Therefore, the purpose of this study was to assess the knowledge about guidelines and procedural considerations in operative dentistry while providing dental care during the COVID-19 pandemic among the DHCPs in the Jazan region of Saudi Arabia. An additional objective of the study was to explore the influence of gender, professional experience, and exposure to guidelines on the level of knowledge among DHCPs. We hypothesised that the level of knowledge among DHCPs would vary across the genders, level of professional experience and exposure to the guidelines.

2. Materials and Methods

2.1. Procedure

A cross-sectional study was conducted 10 months after the onset of the COVID-19 pandemic between January–March 2021 involving DHCP working in the Jazan region. The study was conducted according to the guidelines of the Declaration of Helsinki and approved by the Institutional Review Board of Jazan University (Ref No: CODJU-2028I). A validated questionnaire was circulated online to the participants through emails and various social media platforms.

Information about the study was widely circulated to all dental students, interns and dentists working at Jazan University through emails. An attempt was made to reach out to dentists practising throughout the Jazan region by advertising the study information on social media platforms like Facebook pages, blogs, online forums, and WhatsApp groups on dentistry. The advertising information included the link to the online survey. Those willing to participate provided consent before proceeding to complete the survey. DHCP practising in the Jazan region was only eligible to participate. DHCP who are retired, currently not practising and outside the Jazan region were ineligible to participate.

StatCalc component of the Epi info statistical program was used for sample size calculation [19]. The pilot study's findings indicated that 50% of the subjects had high LOA. With an expected frequency of 50%, an acceptable margin of error of 5%, a confidence level of 95%, and an estimated population size of 2000, the required sample size was 322. A recent study reported 287 public sector oral health care providers in the Jazan region, but we have assumed the population size of all DHCPs in both private and public sectors to be 2000 [20].

Google Forms was used to develop the online survey, composed of three major domains: Informed consent, Demographic characteristics and COVID-19 prevention and control guidelines. The first component explained the intended purpose of the research; participants had to provide consent before answering the survey. No personal identifying information was obtained to maintain confidentiality except the email address to educate the participants with correct responses post-survey and to eliminate the data of those participants later who decided to withdraw from the study.

The face and content validity of the questionnaire was evaluated. The relevance of the questions was reviewed by two content experts from the Department of Restorative Dental Sciences who had thoroughly understood the COVID-19 prevention guidelines. After their approval, the resulting survey was pilot tested on a subset of 25 participants. Some of the items were simplified without changing the content as the participants could not comprehend them. The pilot sample constituted 25 participants (10 dental students, 6 interns and 9 dental practitioners) recruited from the Jazan University dental clinics. The pilot sample has refrained from participation in the main study. The reliability of the questionnaire on repeated administration was estimated by administering the survey to the same 25 participants after a gap of 2 weeks. After eliminating invalid responses, the internal consistency of questions was evaluated.

2.2. Data Collection

Demographic information (gender) and level of professional skills were recorded. Prior to questions targeting knowledge, participants' exposure to dental guidelines and workshops on COVID-19 infection prevention and control was recorded using two items with a dichotomous response of yes/no. Knowledge was evaluated using 35 closed-ended items (Table S1), 29 items (item 1, 3–25, 28, 32–35) were adapted from the collective clinical protocols recommended in a previous systematic review [21]. These recommendations were derived by systematically reviewing the published literature and guidelines laid down by various international healthcare institutions on general dentistry. Six questions relevant to operative dental procedures (items 2, 26, 27, 29, 30, 31) were added. These six items were developed and approved by a panel of four experts from two departments (Restorative and Preventive Dental Sciences). The questions had a five-point Likert scale ranging from 'strongly disagree (score 1)' to 'strongly agree (score 5)'. Eleven questions were negatively worded (items 6, 7, 11, 18, 20, 21, 23, 27, 28, 29, 32) and were subsequently reverse scored, 'strongly disagree (score 5)' to 'strongly agree (score 1)'. Overall knowledge scores were estimated by summing up the item scores, with higher scores indicating better knowledge.

Items 1–20 were related to guidelines to be followed before starting any dental procedures, while items 21–32 were related to guidelines to be followed during the dental procedures, while items 33–35 comprised guidelines to be followed after the dental procedures had been completed. It took approximately 10 min to answer the questionnaire. A participant was considered to provide a correct response when they agreed/strongly agreed to a positive statement or disagreed/strongly disagreed to a negative statement depending upon the intended meaning of the question concerning the corresponding guideline statement.

Based on the responses to the 35 knowledge items, the participant's overall level of awareness (LOA) was assessed. The LOA was classified as high and low based on the number of correct responses; a 75th percentile was used to determine the cut-off. Participants providing 26 or more corrected responses were considered to have high LOA, while the remaining were considered to have low LOA. Awareness of each guideline statement was determined by the participants' frequency and percentage of positive and negative responses.

2.3. Statistical Analysis

The collected data were analysed with the SPSS (Version 23.0; IBM, Chicago, IL, USA) software program. Descriptive statistics were conducted. Chi-square tests were performed to check the association between LOA with gender, level of professional skills, exposure to infection control guidelines and workshops. Frequencies and percentages were used to demonstrate the participants' responses to each item.

An exploratory factor analysis (EFA) was conducted to evaluate the dimensionality of the 35-item questionnaire, principal component analysis with varimax rotation and Kaiser normalisation was used. Scree plot and Kaiser criterion (Eigenvalue > 1) were used to determine component retention. EFA was repeated by restricting the number of factors to be extracted based on the Scree plot and Kaiser criteria [22]. The Factorability of the questionnaire was determined using the Kaiser–Meyer–Olkin (KMO) test and Bartlett's test of sphericity.

A KMO value of ≥ 0.8 with a significant Bartlett test was considered to denote an adequate sample size for factor analysis [23]. Items with factor loadings ≥ 0.30 were considered for inclusion. A cut-off of $\geq$0.30 is considered adequate when the sample size is over 300 [24]. Subscale scores were estimated by summing up the scores of the items in the derived factors. Internal consistency reliability of the overall questionnaire and its factors was evaluated using Cronbach's alpha. A Cronbach's alpha of >0.8 was considered adequate [25]. A split-half test was used to estimate reliability on repeated administration. Means and standard deviations (SD) were estimated for factor scores. Unpaired t-tests were used to compare the factor scores concerning gender and exposure of guidelines, while one way ANOVA was used for professional experience. A p-value of <0.05 was considered statistically significant.

3. Results

Overall, 61.2% of the participants had high LOA (Table 1). A greater number of dentists were found to have high LOA (65.6%) as compared to dental students (62.5%) and interns (46.2%) ($p = 0.0001$). Among 35 guideline statements, more than 50% of the participants were aware of 26 guideline statements. The majority of the respondents (54–90.9%) were unaware of nine guideline statements corresponding to items 6, 11, 21, 23, 26–29 and 32. Of these nine guideline statements, items 6 and 11 belong to the protocols to be followed before the dental procedure, and the remaining items are to be followed during the procedure. More than 50% of the participants were aware of the protocols to be followed after completing the dental procedure (Table 2).

Table 1. Association between levels of awareness with gender, level of professional skills, exposure of guidelines and workshops.

Variable	Level of Awareness *N* (%) Low (n = 141)	High (n = 222)	Total	Chi-Square	*p*-Value
Gender					
Male	79 (36.74)	136 (63.26)	215	0.9780	0.3230
Female	62 (41.89)	86 (58.11)	148		
Level of professional skills					
Practitioners	41 (34.45)	78 (65.55)	119	33.9650	0.0001 *
Students	72 (37.50)	120 (62.50)	192		
Interns	28 (53.85)	24 (46.15)	52		
Exposure to guidelines					
Not read	15 (53.57)	13 (46.43)	28	2.8400	0.0920
Read	126 (37.61)	209 (62.39)	335		
Attendance in workshops					
Not attended	52 (29.55)	124 (70.45)	176	12.4320	0.0001 *
Attended	89 (47.59)	98 (52.41)	187		

* $p < 0.05$.

Table 2. Frequency and percentage of participants' responses to each item.

Item	Strongly Disagree *N* (%)	Disagree *N* (%)	Neutral *N* (%)	Agree *N* (%)	Strongly Agree *N* (%)
1. Patients with non-urgent conditions should be encouraged to maintain proper oral hygiene by consuming a healthy diet, avoiding hard or sticky food, and keeping good oral hygiene practices to preserve their current status.	0 (0)	0 (0)	8 (2.2)	169 (46.6)	186 (51.2)
2. Patients with reversible pulpitis and dentine hypersensitivity should be recommended analgesics if needed, avoid stimuli (cold, hot and acidic drinks or food), apply desensitising toothpaste regularly to the sensitive area with a finger, and advise the patient to call back if symptoms get worse.	6 (1.7)	31 (8.5)	61 (16.8)	155 (42.7)	110 (30.3)
3. Prevent crowding in appointment setting by booking appointments	1 (0.3)	0 (0)	23 (6.3)	120 (33.1)	219 (60.3)
4. Any dental procedures should be delayed in patients with a history of COVID-19 for at least a month	5 (1.4)	35 (9.6)	53 (14.6)	146 (40.2)	124 (34.2)
5. High-risk patients like diabetic and immunocompromised patients should be treated early in a dental office opening.	1 (0.3)	5 (1.4)	73 (20.1)	136 (37.5)	148 (40.7)
6. Telephonic triage/Tele dentistry should not be considered an alternative to in-office care.	30 (8.3)	35 (9.6)	154 (42.4)	69 (19.0)	75 (20.7)
7. Patients with fracture/loose tooth fragments or broken restorations should be referred to the designated urgent dental clinics during the COVID-19 pandemic.	11 (3.0)	28 (7.7)	93 (25.6)	137 (37.7)	94 (25.9)

Table 2. *Cont.*

Item	Strongly Disagree N (%)	Disagree N (%)	Neutral N (%)	Agree N (%)	Strongly Agree N (%)
8. The temperature of staff and patients should be monitored daily	2 (0.6)	2 (0.6)	16 (4.4)	70 (19.3)	273 (75.2)
9. Ask dental health care personnel to stay home if they are sick	0 (0)	2 (0.6)	17 (4.7)	91 (25.1)	253 (69.7)
10. Patients with fever should be referred to a specific medical centre treating COVID-19	8 (2.2)	7 (1.9)	31 (8.5)	128 (35.3)	189 (52.1)
11. Accompanying individuals with patients should be allowed in the clinics.	79 (21.8)	88 (24.2)	85 (23.4)	81 (22.3)	30 (8.3)
12. Hand disinfection with 60–75% alcohol should be offered upon entrance to the dental office.	2 (0.6)	1 (0.3)	33 (9.1)	149 (41.1)	178 (49.0)
13. Emergency dental care can be provided if a patient's temperature is less than 100.4-degrees Fahrenheit and does not have symptoms consistent with COVID-19.	5 (1.4)	31 (8.5)	90 (24.8)	160 (44.1)	77 (21.2)
14. The waiting area should be large with adequate ventilation.	0 (0)	28 (7.7)	13 (3.6)	89 (24.5)	233 (64.2)
15. The 2-m separation between patients is mandatory in waiting rooms and reception areas.	0 (0)	2 (0.6)	47 (13.0)	98 (27.0)	216 (59.5)
16. Remove magazines, toys, and other objects which cannot be easily disinfected	0 (0)	29 (8.0)	44 (12.1)	84 (23.1)	206 (56.8)
17. Posters in the dental office for instructing patients on standard recommendations for respiratory hygiene/cough etiquette and social distancing should be posted in appropriate places.	0 (0)	0 (0)	29 (8.0)	160 (44.1)	174 (48.0)
18. It is not required by everyone entering the dental office to use facemasks or cloth face coverings.	133 (36.6)	81 (22.3)	41 (11.3)	77 (21.2)	31 (8.5)
19. Dental procedures require professionals to use Personal protective equipment (surgical caps, gloves, N-95 mask, FFP2 mask, goggles, gowns, and face shields).	0 (0)	6 (1.7)	39 (10.7)	112 (30.8)	206 (56.8)
20. It is not required to cover all touchable surfaces with disposable protections.	108 (29.8)	80 (22.0)	93 (25.6)	53 (14.6)	29 (8.0)
21. Patients should not be treated in rooms with negative pressure relative to the surrounding area.	12 (3.3)	21 (5.8)	119 (32.8)	160 (44.1)	51 (14.1)
22. In case hands are visibly soiled, water and soap should be used at least 20 s before using an Alcohol-based hand rub.	3 (0.8)	8 (2.2)	29 (8.0)	186 (51.2)	137 (37.7)
23. Preprocedural mouth rinse like 1.5% hydrogen peroxide or 0.2% povidone should not be used before starting any dental procedure in the patient.	40 (11.0)	54 (14.9)	120 (33.1)	79 (21.8)	70 (19.3)

Table 2. *Cont.*

Item	Strongly Disagree N (%)	Disagree N (%)	Neutral N (%)	Agree N (%)	Strongly Agree N (%)
24. Avoid the use of topical spray anaesthesia to prevent gag reflex	10 (2.8)	32 (8.8)	132 (36.4)	156 (43.0)	33 (9.1)
25. Use of rubber dam and N-95 masks are mandatory for aerosol-generating dental procedures	1 (0.3)	23(6.3)	47 (13.0)	124 (34.2)	168 (46.3)
26. High-volume saliva ejectors can increase aerosol or spatter while performing dental procedures	61 (16.8)	55 (15.2)	63 (17.4)	142 (39.1)	42 (11.6)
27. Panoramic radiographs or cone-beam computed tomographs should not be used for intraoral radiography	31 (8.5)	87 (24.0)	103 (28.4)	68 (18.7)	74 (20.4)
28. Four-handed dentistry should not be practised for aerosol-generating procedures.	36 (9.9)	78 (21.5)	124 (34.2)	69 (19.0)	56 (15.4)
29. Use of 3-in-1 syringes, air-water syringes, and ultrasonic instruments are allowed for all aerosol-generating dental procedures	24 (6.6)	45 (12.4)	125 (34.4)	136 (37.5)	33 (9.1)
30. Adopt the Atraumatic Restorative Technique and Chemo mechanical caries removal procedure wherever possible	0 (0)	14 (3.9)	92 (25.3)	154 (42.4)	103 (28.4)
31. To reduce the clinical time, preferences should be given to bulk-fill composite resin restorations as it permits increments up to 4 mm in thickness.	24 (6.6)	61 (16.8)	95 (26.2)	118 (32.5)	65 (18.0)
32. Treatment should be completed in multiple visits wherever possible.	60 (16.5)	68 (18.7)	83 (22.9)	119 (32.8)	33 (9.1)
33. Environmental cleaning and disinfection procedures should be followed after completion of treatment	2 (0.6)	0 (0)	45 (12.4)	124 (34.2)	192 (52.9)
34. Clean and disinfect reusable PPE	12 (3.3)	27 (7.4)	58 (16.0)	111 (30.6)	155 (42.7)
35. Manage laundry and medical waste following routine procedures	11 (3.0)	8 (2.2)	40 (11.0)	160 (44.1)	144 (39.7)

Among the six guideline statements related to operative dentistry (item 2, 26, 28, 29, 30, 31), more than 50% of the participants were aware of items 2, 30 and 31. Furthermore, awareness of the remaining 3 guideline statements was less than 50%.

EFA demonstrated that the KMO value was 0.86, and Bartlett's test of sphericity was significant ($p < 0.001$), indicating sampling adequacy. Three distinct factors were derived from the EFA. Factor loadings are presented in Table 3, and all the items had factor loadings of >0.3 except one item, "Any dental procedures should be delayed in patients with a history of COVID-19 for at least a month", that had a loading of 0.28. As the item was closely related to factor 3, it was included in factor 3. The Cronbach's value of the overall scale with 35 items was 0.81, while factors 1, 2 and 3 had a Cronbach's alpha of 0.87, 0.85 and 0.82, respectively. Reliability on repeated administration was assessed using split-half reliability, and it was 0.91. Table 4 demonstrates that males had significantly higher scores on all the factors than females. Those who have not attended workshops had significantly higher scores for factors 2 and 3 than those who attended ($p < 0.05$).

Table 3. Factor loadings of the 35 items.

Item	Factor 1	Factor 2	Factor 3
	Guidelines Related to Dental Treatment Procedures	Guidelines Related to General COVID-19 Cross-Infection Control Procedures	Guidelines Related to Maintenance of Waiting Areas and Appointments/Referrals
Four-handed dentistry should not be practised for aerosol-generating procedures.	0.75		
Accompanying individuals with patients should be allowed in the clinics.	0.72		
It is not required to cover all touchable surfaces with disposable protections.	0.71		
It is not required by everyone entering the dental office to use facemasks or cloth face coverings.	0.70		
Use of 3-in-1 syringes, air-water syringes, and ultrasonic instruments are allowed for all aerosol-generating dental procedures	0.67		
Preprocedural mouth rinse like 1.5% hydrogen peroxide or 0.2% povidone should not be used before starting any dental procedure in the patient.	0.66		
Treatment should be completed in multiple visits wherever possible.	0.65		
High-volume saliva ejectors can increase aerosol or spatter while performing dental procedures.	0.65		
Patients should not be treated in rooms with negative pressure relative to the surrounding area.	0.61		
Panoramic radiographs or cone-beam computed tomographs should not be used for intraoral radiography.	0.53		
Telephonic triage/Tele dentistry should not be considered an alternate option to in-office care.	0.50		
Avoid the use of topical spray anaesthesia to prevent gag reflex	0.49		
To reduce the clinical time, preferences should be given to bulk-fill composite resin restorations as it permits increments up to 4 mm in thickness.	0.36		
Patients with reversible pulpitis and dentine hypersensitivity should be recommended analgesics if needed, avoid stimuli (cold, hot and acidic drinks or food), apply desensitising toothpaste regularly to the sensitive area with a finger, and advise the patient to call back if symptoms get worse	0.31		
Use of rubber dam and N-95 masks are mandatory for aerosol-generating dental procedures		0.72	
Environmental cleaning and disinfection procedures should be followed after completion of treatment		0.68	
The temperature of staff and patients should be monitored daily		0.66	
Adopt the Atraumatic Restorative Technique and Chemo mechanical caries removal procedure wherever possible		0.65	
Ask dental health care personnel to stay home if they are sick		0.64	
Dental procedures require professionals to use Personal protective equipment (surgical caps, gloves, N-95 mask, FFP2 mask, goggles, gowns, and face shields).		0.60	
Clean and disinfect reusable PPE		0.56	
Patients with fever should be referred to a specific medical centre treating COVID-19		0.54	
Hand disinfection with 60–75% alcohol should be offered upon entrance to the dental office.		0.50	

Table 3. *Cont.*

Item	Factor 1	Factor 2	Factor 3
	Guidelines Related to Dental Treatment Procedures	Guidelines Related to General COVID-19 Cross-Infection Control Procedures	Guidelines Related to Maintenance of Waiting Areas and Appointments/Referrals
In case hands are visibly soiled, water and soap should be used at least 20 s before using an Alcohol-based hand rub.		0.49	
Manage laundry and medical waste following routine procedures		0.40	
The waiting area should be large with adequate ventilation			0.80
The 2-m separation between patients is mandatory in waiting rooms and reception areas.			0.72
Remove magazines, toys, and other objects which cannot be easily disinfected			0.72
High-risk patients like diabetic and immunocompromised patients should be treated in the early hours of a dental office opening.			0.65
Posters in the dental office for instructing patients on standard recommendations for respiratory hygiene/cough etiquette and social distancing should be posted in appropriate places.			0.56
Patients with non-urgent conditions should be encouraged to maintain proper oral hygiene by consuming a healthy diet, avoiding hard or sticky food, and keeping good oral hygiene practices to preserve their current status.			0.56
Patients with fracture/loose tooth fragments or broken restorations should be referred to the designated urgent dental clinics during the COVID-19 pandemic.			0.51
Emergency dental care can be provided if a patient's temperature is less than 100.4-degrees Fahrenheit and does not have symptoms consistent with COVID-19.			0.43
Prevent crowding in appointment settings by booking appointments			0.40
Any dental procedures should be delayed in patients with a history of COVID-19 for at least a month *			0.28

* loading < 0.30.

Table 4. Overall and factor scores concerning gender, level of professional skills, exposure to guidelines and workshops.

Variable		Guidelines Related to Dental Treatment Procedures Mean (SD)	Guidelines Related to General COVID-19 Cross-Infection Control Procedures Mean (SD)	Guidelines Related to Maintenance of Waiting Areas and Appointments/Referrals Mean (SD)
Gender	Males	45.64 (9.72) *	46.88 (5.95) *	41.50 (5.63) *
	Females	42.27 (9.87)	48.14 (5.02)	43.35 (4.12)
Level of professional skills	Practitioners	45.39 (10.70) †	47.47 (5.80)	41.53 (6.41) †
	Students	44.53 (9.48)	47.80 (5.02)	43.01 (3.98)
	Interns	40.73 (8.89)	45.73 (6.97)	41.15 (5.37)
Exposure to guidelines	Not read	46.64 (11.40)	44.89 (4.60) *	41.18 (4.92)
	Read	44.07 (9.76)	47.60 (5.65)	42.35 (5.16)
Attendance of workshops	Not attended	44.38 (9.70)	48.66 (4.77) *	43.60 (3.89) *
	Attended	44.16 (10.13)	46.20 (6.09)	40.99 (5.82)

* Unpaired *t*-test, $p < 0.05$; † one-way ANOVA, $p < 0.05$.

4. Discussion

Documents relevant to COVID-19 infection guidelines have been released by various organisations worldwide [2,4,5,13,14]. As and when these guidance documents are periodically updated, it is the moral and ethical responsibility of the dental care health workers to be updated to prevent the spread and contain the pandemic. A survey from Turkey showed that 1.8% (n = 17) of the participant dentists were positively tested against COVID-19, highlighting the increased risk for dental professionals [26]. The current study was conducted to check the awareness of COVID-19 infection prevention and control guidelines recommended by various governing organisations before, during, and after performing dental procedures among dental students, interns, and dentists in the Jazan region of Saudi Arabia.

Various studies have been conducted to check the knowledge, attitudes, and practices of COVID-19 infection prevention among dental students, interns, and dentists in Saudi Arabia [12,26,27]. Stratifying the participants based on their level of professional experience was done to investigate the difference in awareness. However, we did not find any study that evaluated the awareness of a comprehensive set of COVID-19 infection prevention and control guidelines. In addition, we developed the survey adopting the questions from previous studies and evaluated the questionnaire's validity and reliability. The questionnaire was reliable and valid, with three distinct factors demonstrating that researchers within and outside Saudi Arabia could use it.

The response rate of similar studies conducted in Saudi Arabia was 28.7% [28], 28.2% [29] and 21.7% [30]. These values are much lower than our study's response rate of 60.5%, probably due to variation in the target population. In this study, it was found that a majority (92.29%) of the participants read the guidelines for providing dental services during the COVID-19 pandemic. There was no significant difference or association between respondents who read and did not read the guidelines of COVID-19 with LOA. This could be due to the constant update on COVID-19 infection guidelines by national and international bodies through different media.

Moreover, it was revealed in the study that only half of the participants had attended COVID-19 infection prevention workshops. However, surprisingly, fewer participants who attended the workshops had high LOA and were more aware of guidelines related to general COVID-19 cross-infection prevention and precautions in the waiting area than those who did not attend COVID-19 infection prevention workshops. This might be due to the ever-changing/updating of the guidelines as the pandemic has been evolving. DHCPs who have attended workshops might have been complacent, assuming that the workshops they have attended have provided them with comprehensive information. On the other hand, those respondents who have not participated in the workshops might constantly be making themselves aware of the evolving guidelines. It appears that the workshops conducted are not emphasising the international guidelines.

The dentists in the present study have a significantly higher level of awareness than students and interns, particularly guidelines related to preventing cross-infection in the operatory and waiting room. These findings are consistent with a study conducted among Turkish dental professionals that revealed higher knowledge about the COVID-19 aetiology, mode of transmission and the pre-procedural cautions among dental specialist respondents. These findings indicate a direct correlation between professional experience and LOA which is in total agreement with the previous studies [12,31] and disagreement with other studies reported from in Saudi Arabia [28] and Jordan [28,32]. The variation in LOA could be attributed to the difference in perception and education of the DHCP.

None of the participants in the Jazan region had poor LOA. Similar results have been reported in various studies conducted in Saudi Arabia, where the basic knowledge on COVID-19 among the DHCP was satisfactory and acceptable [12,26]. This can be attributed to the Saudi MOH's extensive efforts to educate the DHCP about the pandemic outbreak and the associated risk of transmission. A study conducted among dental students and interns in different universities of Cairo, Egypt, revealed that they also had good knowledge and awareness about COVID-19 and the necessary precautions required to provide adequate dental treatment for the patients during the pandemic COVID-19 [33].

Among 35 guideline statements, more than 50% of participants were aware of 26 guidelines, while awareness was less than 50% for the remaining nine guideline statements. These findings are consistent with a global study that evaluated the level of knowledge and the attitude of dental practitioners related to disinfection during the COVID-19 pandemic, which indicated that the respondents did not have complete knowledge to implement disinfection guidelines specifically against COVID-19 [34]. The majority (97.8%) of participants were aware that all non-urgent conditions could be delayed by encouraging the patient to maintain proper oral hygiene. It could be attributed to the fact that the DHCP is scared and anxious in handling patients suspected of COVID-19 infection [35]. Interestingly, participants were unaware of nine guideline items (two related to the protocols to be followed before the dental procedure, and the remaining items are to be followed during the procedure). Hence, it is recommended to educate the DHCP on those guidelines before and during the dental procedure to ensure the safety and prevention of COVID-19 cross-infection.

In this study, it was alarming to know that more than 90% of the respondents were unaware of the recommendation that dental patients should be treated in rooms with negative pressure relative to the surrounding area [2,5,13,14] Similarly, 82.1% of the respondents were not aware that telephonic triage was recommended during the COVID-19 pandemic [2,5,13,14] This could be attributed to the reason that most of our survey respondents were working within university or MOH clinic sectors and not private practices. Those aspects are handled by public relations teams instead of DHCP in such facilities.

Among the items about operative dentistry, most (80%) of the respondents were unaware that during the COVID-19 pandemic, it is not recommended to use 3-in-1 syringes and ultrasonic instruments (item 29) while performing AGPs [2,5,13,15,16]. Furthermore, many (68%) respondents were unaware that four-handed dentistry (item 28) and high-volume saliva ejectors (item 26) are recommended for AGPs [2,13,16,17]. Since operative dentistry constitutes a significant part of the dental practice, the DHCP must concentrate on these guideline statements to preclude the spread of COVID-19 infection.

Based on our findings, to encourage the reading of guidelines, exams must be conducted to check the awareness of guidelines among students and interns before allowing them to work independently on patients. New evidence-based guidelines should be displayed as posters in appropriate clinical areas and posted on various social media platforms targeting the DHCPs. To increase the awareness of COVID-19 among the general masses and persuade them to follow guidelines, the government of Bhutan engaged actors, bloggers, visual artists and sports personalities [36]. Similarly, social media influencers can be hired to inform and influence the DHCPs, especially the students and interns. In addition, video resources that provide comprehensive information on the infection control procedures and sequences could be developed, similar to those developed by the Australian dental association, to demonstrate the donning and doffing sequences of the PPE [37].

The DHCPs should be reminded of the significance of doing clinical procedures in unfavourable pressure rooms, utilising large volume saliva ejectors, avoiding using 3-in-1 syringes, air-water syringes, or ultrasonic tools, and practising four-handed dentistry [2,5,13,15–17]. Methods such as bio-inspired systems should be adopted while performing dental procedures because these systems are showing promising results in reducing bacteremia and aerosol generation, improving immunological, microbiological, and clinical parameters [38].

This study was conducted among self-selected DHCP in the Jazan region of Saudi Arabia; therefore, the findings could not be generalised to DHCP throughout the country, and a larger sample size would yield a more precise overview of DHCP awareness. Nevertheless, the aim was to analyse the subjects in the Jazan region alone.

5. Conclusions

The majority of DHCP had high LOA regarding the general guidelines related to infection prevention and control of COVID-19. As far as the guidelines related to operative dentistry procedures are concerned, most DHCP was unaware that during the COVID-19 pandemic, a three-way syringe has to be avoided, four-handed dentistry should be practised, and high-volume saliva ejectors should be used during AGPs. Dentists, males, and those who read the guidelines had higher LOA than their counterparts. Based on our research findings, it is recommended to conduct lectures and seminars related to COVID-19 infection prevention control guidelines to all DHCPs in general and students and interns in particular. A task force should be organised at the institutional level to provide consolidated evidence-based guidelines and updates for all DHCPs.

Supplementary Materials: The following supporting information can be downloaded at: https://www.mdpi.com/article/10.3390/ijerph19042034/s1, Table S1: Questionnaire.

Author Contributions: Conceptualisation, S.N.B., T.S.V. and M.I.K.; methodology, N.H.M.A., S.K.T.; software, A.R. and L.M.A.; validation, M.I.K. and A.B.; formal analysis, S.W.P. and S.A.P.; investigation, S.N.B. and T.S.V.; resources, M.I.K. and N.H.M.A.; data curation, S.N.B. and T.S.V.; writing—original draft preparation S.N.B. and T.S.V.; writing—review and editing, M.I.K. and S.K.T.; visualisation, S.W.P. and S.A.P.; supervision, S.N.B., M.I.K. and S.K.T.; project administration, S.N.B. and T.S.V.; funding acquisition, A.R. and T.S.V. All authors have read and agreed to the published version of the manuscript.

Funding: This research received no external funding.

Institutional Review Board Statement: The study was conducted according to the guidelines of the Declaration of Helsinki and approved by the Institutional Review of Jazan University (Ref No: CODJU-2028I).

Informed Consent Statement: Informed consent was obtained from all subjects involved in the study.

Data Availability Statement: The data set used in the current study will be made available at a reasonable request.

Conflicts of Interest: The authors declare no conflict of interest.

References

1. Cao, W.; Li, T. COVID-19: Towards understanding of pathogenesis. *Cell Res.* **2020**, *30*, 367–369. [CrossRef] [PubMed]
2. CDC. Centers for Disease Control and Prevention. Interim Infection Prevention and Control Guidance for Dental Settings during the COVID-19 Response. Available online: https://www.cdc.gov/coronavirus/2019-ncov/hcp/dental-settings.html (accessed on 1 February 2022).
3. WHO. Corona Virus (COVID-19) Dashboard. Available online: https://covid19.who.int/ (accessed on 1 February 2022).
4. WHO. World Health Organization. Coronavirus Disease (COVID-19) Technical Guidance: Infection Prevention and Control/WASH, WHO. Available online: https://www.who.int/emergencies/diseases/novel-coronavirus-2019/technical-guidance/infection-prevention-and-control (accessed on 1 February 2022).
5. MOH. COVID-19 Guidelines. Available online: https://www.moh.gov.sa/en/Ministry/MediaCenter/Publications/Pages/covid19.aspx (accessed on 1 February 2022).
6. Peng, X.; Xu, X.; Li, Y.; Cheng, L.; Zhou, X.; Ren, B. Transmission routes of 2019-nCoV and controls in dental practice. *Int. J. Oral Sci.* **2020**, *12*, 9. [CrossRef] [PubMed]
7. Meng, L.; Hua, F.; Bian, Z. Coronavirus Disease 2019 (COVID-19): Emerging and Future Challenges for Dental and Oral Medicine. *J. Dent. Res.* **2020**, *99*, 481–487. [CrossRef] [PubMed]
8. Van Doremalen, N.; Bushmaker, T.; Morris, D.H.; Holbrook, M.G.; Gamble, A.; Williamson, B.N.; Tamin, A.; Harcourt, J.L.; Thornburg, N.J.; Gerber, S.I.; et al. Aerosol and Surface Stability of SARS-CoV-2 as Compared with SARS-CoV-1. *N. Engl. J. Med.* **2020**, *382*, 1564–1567. [CrossRef]
9. Froum, S.H.; Froum, S.J. Incidence of COVID-19 Virus Transmission in Three Dental Offices: A 6-Month Retrospective Study. *Int. J. Periodontics Restor. Dent.* **2020**, *40*, 853–859. [CrossRef]
10. Halim, M.S.; Noorani, T.Y.; Karobari, M.I.; Kamaruddin, N. COVID-19 and dental education: A Malaysian perspective. *J. Int. Oral Health* **2021**, *13*, 201.
11. Basheer, S.N.; Peeran, S.W.; Peeran, S.A.; Zameer, M.; Naviwala, G.A.; Elhassan, A.T. Knowledge, attitude and practices of health-care professionals related to COVID-19: A multi country survey. *Dent. Med. Res.* **2021**, *9*, 100.

12. Quadri, M.F.A.; Jafer, M.A.; Alqahtani, A.S.; Al mutahar, S.A.B.; Odabi, N.I.; Daghriri, A.A.; Tadakamadla, S.K. Novel corona virus disease (COVID-19) awareness among the dental interns, dental auxiliaries and dental specialists in Saudi Arabia: A nationwide study. *J. Infect. Public Health* **2020**, *13*, 856–864. [CrossRef]
13. ADA. American Dental Association Guidelines, Infectious-Diseases-2019-Novel-Coronavirus. Available online: https://success.ada.org/en/practice-management/patients/infectious-diseases-2019-novel-coronavirus (accessed on 1 February 2022).
14. NHS. Scottish Dental Clinical Effectiveness Programme, Resources for COVID-19. Available online: https://www.sdcep.org.uk (accessed on 1 February 2022).
15. Ather, A.; Patel, B.; Ruparel, N.B.; Diogenes, A.; Hargreaves, K.M. Reply to "Coronavirus Disease 19 (COVID-19): Implications for Clinical Dental Care". *J. Endod.* **2020**, *46*, 1342. [CrossRef]
16. Izzetti, R.; Nisi, M.; Gabriele, M.; Graziani, F. COVID-19 Transmission in Dental Practice: Brief Review of Preventive Measures in Italy. *J. Dent. Res.* **2020**, *99*, 1030–1038. [CrossRef]
17. Lee, Y.H.; Auh, Q.S. Strategies for prevention of coronavirus disease 2019 in the dental field. *Oral Dis.* **2020**, *27*, 740–741. [CrossRef] [PubMed]
18. Christensen, G.J. CHAPTER 18—Restorative or Operative Dentistry: Fillings for Teeth. In *A Consumer's Guide to Dentistry*, 2nd ed.; Christensen, G.J., Ed.; Mosby: Burlington, NJ, USA, 2002; pp. 167–175. [CrossRef]
19. CDC. Epi Info™, Division of Health Informatics & Surveillance (DHIS), Center for Surveillance, Epidemiology & Laboratory Services (CSELS). Available online: https://www.cdc.gov/epiinfo/user-guide/statcalc/statcalcintro.html (accessed on 25 January 2022).
20. Shubayr, M.A.; Kruger, E.; Tennant, M. Assessment of dental healthcare services and workforce in the Jazan Region, Saudi Arabia. *Saudi J. Oral Dent. Res.* **2021**, *6*, 81–87. [CrossRef]
21. Banakar, M.; Lankarani, K.B.; Jafarpour, D.; Moayedi, S.; Banakar, M.H.; Mohammad Sadeghi, A. COVID-19 transmission risk and protective protocols in dentistry: A systematic review. *BMC Oral Health* **2020**, *20*, 275. [CrossRef] [PubMed]
22. Braeken, J.; Van Assen, M.A. An empirical Kaiser criterion. *Psychol. Methods* **2017**, *22*, 450–466. [CrossRef] [PubMed]
23. Field, A. *Discovering Statistics Using SPSS*; Sage Publications: Sauzende Oaks, CA, USA, 2009.
24. Hair, J.; Black, W.C.; Babin, B.; Anderson, R.; Tatham, R. Pearson new international edition. In *Multivariate Data Analysis*, 7th ed.; Pearson Education Limited: Essex, UK, 2014.
25. Cronbach, L.J. Coefficient alpha and the internal structure of tests. *Psychometrika* **1951**, *16*, 297–334. [CrossRef]
26. Mustafa, R.M.; Alshali, R.Z.; Bukhary, D.M. Dentists' Knowledge, Attitudes, and Awareness of Infection Control Measures during COVID-19 Outbreak: A Cross-Sectional Study in Saudi Arabia. *Int. J. Environ. Res. Public Health* **2020**, *17*, 9016. [CrossRef]
27. Srivastava, K.C.; Shrivastava, D.; Sghaireen, M.G.; Alsharari, A.F.; Alduraywish, A.A.; Al-Johani, K.; Alam, M.K.; Khader, Y.; Alzarea, B.K. Knowledge, attitudes and practices regarding COVID-19 among dental health care professionals: A cross-sectional study in Saudi Arabia. *J. Int. Med. Res.* **2020**, *48*, 300060520977593. [CrossRef]
28. Tarakji, B.; Nassani, M.Z.; Alali, F.M.; Alsalhani, A.B.; Alqhtani, N.R.; Bin Nabhan, A.; Alenzi, A.; Alrafedah, A. COVID-19—awareness and practice of dentists in Saudi Arabia. *Int. J. Environ. Res. Public Health* **2021**, *18*, 330. [CrossRef]
29. Al-Khalifa, K.S.; AlSheikh, R.; Al-Swuailem, A.S.; Alkhalifa, M.S.; Al-Johani, M.H.; Al-Moumen, S.A.; Almomen, Z.I. Pandemic preparedness of dentists against coronavirus disease: A Saudi Arabian experience. *PLoS ONE* **2020**, *15*, e0237630. [CrossRef]
30. Shahin, S.Y.; Bugshan, A.S.; Almulhim, K.S.; AlSharief, M.S.; Al-Dulaijan, Y.A.; Siddiqui, I.; Al-Qarni, F.D. Knowledge of dentists, dental auxiliaries, and students regarding the COVID-19 pandemic in Saudi Arabia: A cross-sectional survey. *BMC Oral Health* **2020**, *20*, 1–8. [CrossRef]
31. Karayürek, F.; Yilmaz Çırakoğlu, N.; Gülses, A.; Ayna, M. Awareness and Knowledge of SARS-CoV-2 Infection among Dental Professionals According to the Turkish National Dental Guidelines. *Int. J. Environ. Res. Public Health* **2021**, *18*, 442. [CrossRef] [PubMed]
32. Khader, Y.; Al Nsour, M.; Al-Batayneh, O.B.; Saadeh, R.; Bashier, H.; Alfaqih, M.; Al-Azzam, S.; AlShurman, B.A. Dentists' Awareness, Perception, and Attitude Regarding COVID-19 and Infection Control: Cross-Sectional Study Among Jordanian Dentists. *JMIR Public Health Surveill.* **2020**, *6*, e18798. [CrossRef] [PubMed]
33. Sharaf, R.F.; Kabel, N. Awareness and knowledge of undergraduate dental students about the signs and symptoms of Corona viral infection (COVID-19), and the required infection control measures to prevent its spread. *Bull. Natl. Res. Cent.* **2021**, *45*, 32. [CrossRef] [PubMed]
34. Sarfaraz, S.; Shabbir, J.; Mudasser, M.A.; Khurshid, Z.; Al-Quraini, A.A.A.; Abbasi, M.S.; Ratnayake, J.; Zafar, M.S. Knowledge and Attitude of Dental Practitioners Related to Disinfection during the COVID-19 Pandemic. *Healthcare* **2020**, *8*, 232. [CrossRef] [PubMed]
35. Khan, A.M.; Nawabi, S.; Javed, M.Q. *Dental Faculty's Knowledge and Attitude Regarding COVID-19 Disease in Qassim, Saudi Arabia*; Research Square AJE LLC: Dehan, NC, USA, 2020.
36. MOH. Update: "Our Gyenkhu". Available online: https://www.moh.gov.bt/update-our-gyenkhu-6/ (accessed on 25 January 2022).
37. Sotomayor-Castillo, C.; Li, C.; Kaufman-Francis, K.; Nahidi, S.; Walsh, L.J.; Liberali, S.A.; Irving, E.; Holden, A.C.; Shaban, R.Z. Australian dentists' knowledge, preparedness, and experiences during the COVID-19 pandemic. *Infect. Dis. Health* **2021**, *27*, 49–57. [CrossRef] [PubMed]
38. Butera, A.; Maiorani, C.; Natoli, V.; Bruni, A.; Coscione, C.; Magliano, G.; Giacobbo, G.; Morelli, A.; Moressa, S.; Scribante, A. Bio-Inspired Systems in Nonsurgical Periodontal Therapy to Reduce Contaminated Aerosol during COVID-19: A Comprehensive and Bibliometric Review. *J. Clin. Med.* **2020**, *9*, 3914. [CrossRef] [PubMed]

International Journal of
Environmental Research and Public Health

MDPI

Article

LinguAPP: An m-Health Application for Teledentistry Diagnostics

Matia Fazio [1], Christian Lombardo [2], Giuseppe Marino [1], Anand Marya [3,4], Pietro Messina [2], Giuseppe Alessandro Scardina [2,*], Antonino Tocco [1], Francesco Torregrossa [5] and Cesare Valenti [1,*]

1 Department of Mathematics and Informatics, University of Palermo, 90123 Palermo, Italy; matia.fazio@gmail.com (M.F.); peppe98.marino@gmail.com (G.M.); entonytocco@gmail.com (A.T.)
2 Department of Surgical Oncological and Stomatological Disciplines, University of Palermo, 90133 Palermo, Italy; christianlombardo778@gmail.com (C.L.); pietro.messina01@unipa.it (P.M.)
3 Center for Transdisciplinary Research, Saveetha Dental College, Saveetha Institute of Medical and Technical Science, Saveetha University, Chennai 600077, India; amarya@puthisastra.edu.kh
4 Department of Orthodontics, Faculty of Dentistry, University of Puthisastra, Phnom Penh 12211, Cambodia
5 Department of Informatics, King's College London, London WC2R 2LS, UK; d.ftorregrossa@gmail.com
* Correspondence: alessandro.scardina@unipa.it (G.A.S.); cesare.valenti@unipa.it (C.V.)

Abstract: An Android/iOS application for low-cost mobile devices to aid in dental diagnosis through questionnaire and photos is presented in this paper. The main purposes of our app lie in the ease of use even for nonexperienced users, in the limited hardware requirements that allow a wide diffusion, and in the possibility to modify the questionnaire for different pathologies. This tool was developed in about a month at the beginning of the COVID-19 (SARS-CoV-2) pandemic and is still in use in Italy to allow support to patients without going to the hospital, if not strictly necessary.

Keywords: dentistry diagnostics; m-health application; medical questionnaire; teledentistry

Citation: Fazio, M.; Lombardo, C.; Marino, G.; Marya, A.; Messina, P.; Scardina, G.A.; Tocco, A.; Torregrossa, F.; Valenti, C. LinguAPP: An m-Health Application for Teledentistry Diagnostics. *Int. J. Environ. Res. Public Health* **2022**, *19*, 822. https://doi.org/10.3390/ijerph19020822

Academic Editors: Paul B. Tchounwou and Hiroko Miura

Received: 9 December 2021
Accepted: 5 January 2022
Published: 12 January 2022

1. Introduction

Recently, m-health applications (i.e., medicine supported by mobile devices) have been applied to various medical fields due to the wide diffusion of mobile devices, the low cost of Internet connection, and the ability to reach substantially almost any remote area [1,2]. Systems to perform an initial diagnosis automatically have been presented in the literature, but a comparison with a medical specialist who provides the final indications and therapy is always appropriate [3,4]. Machine learning for the triage of skin lesions was proposed in [5], while artificial intelligence for ophthalmic screening is described in a broad sense in [6]. Sometimes the use of additional hardware is required to enhance the optics or lighten the computational load on the mobile device [7–11]. A general review of a variety of m-health applications for chronic conditions and/or diseases is given in [12], while COVID-19 (SARS-CoV-2) teledentistry opportunities are described in [13,14].

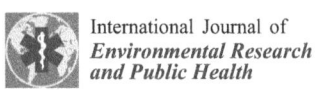

During the early stages of the current COVID-19 pandemic condition, we needed to develop, in a very tight time constraint, a mobile device app to provide medical staff with useful dental information. A further fundamental requirement was the need not to use any additional hardware and to take full advantage of the features of entry-level cell phones. This allowed to give immediate assistance to the population and to arrange an eventual dedicated hospital intervention, avoiding dangerous contact with the rest of the hospitalized patients. Our app, called LinguApp, is freely downloadable for Android and iOS operating systems and is still in use at the Department of Surgical Oncological and Stomatological Disciplines in Palermo, Italy, even though it provides support for the entire country of Italy. This tool submits a triage questionnaire, formulated in a simple way for nonspecialists, and prompts them to take at least two photos to highlight lesions within their mouth without the use of any template to refer. The specialist is then contacted through an e-mail and can provide a preliminary diagnosis by means of a web interface. One of the main advantages of this application lies in the simplicity with which the questionnaire can be managed through the same interface. This feature allows LinguApp to be modified so that after the COVID-19 emergency, it is aimed directly at medical specialists with a more complete and unfamiliar questionnaire, translated into different languages and used in different contexts that can benefit from a questionnaire with attached photos and videos.

In the field of oral pathologies, it is fundamental to make a diagnosis [15,16]: through (*dia*) knowledge (*gnosis*), we aim to answer the question: What is the patient suffering from? In order to have enough knowledge to allow to name a wound, it is necessary to understand the visited patient: lifestyle habits, assumption of drugs, presence of systemic pathologies (generalized or localized), familiarity for certain medical conditions, history of the lesion in the matter, related markers, and symptoms are all aspects that will have to be collected and connected to each other to allow a diagnostic suspicion [17]. This suspicion will be confirmed with the help of any instrumental/histological/microbiological/hematological/clinical examinations [18–20]. Consequently, the diagnosis requires the acquisition of certain information essential for the understanding of the clinical condition of the patient.

The objective of this study is the development of a mobile application to gather the first piece of information for the diagnosis. This application does not have any diagnostic confirmation purpose, which remains exclusively for the objective and instrumental examination in presence, but allows to start a diagnostic path in line with the indications and directives during the quarantine due to COVID-19. Considering the high risk of viral contagion by airborne propagation that dental procedures have inherent in their specificity, these organizations suggest to limit all dental examinations in presence with the exception of urgency and absolute non-deference. During the first pandemic period (in Italy, approximately in March and April 2019), there was the deontological indication to limit treatments only in the case of urgent and unavoidable emergencies, suggesting remote consultation, video consulting, and specialist advice by phone. By using LinguApp on any Android or iOS mobile device, the patient describes his/her symptoms, takes some pictures, and sends all the data directly to a team of specialists who evaluate the actual need to refer the patient to highly specialized centers. Our application is intended mainly for immobilized and noncooperative patients in difficult locations who cannot go to medical facilities during this emergency period [17].

The ability to distinguish one lesion from another is not always so simple, nor so fast. We designed an interactive procedure to navigate a directed graph that helps us identify various lesions hypothetically detectable, in relation to the soft tissues of the oral cavity. The app imposes an order of questions to be answered unambiguously: in this way, the questions divide the large group of "mouth lesions" into smaller, different groups, allowing us to reach a diagnosis of presumption by evaluating the attached photos.

2. Methods

To solve the problem, among the possible viable implementations, the choice fell on the development of two distinct products: a mobile application aimed at patients, and a dashboard or content management system aimed at clinicians.

The choice, on the patients' side, was dictated by the widespread diffusion that smartphones have had in recent years, due to their typically low cost and ease of use that result from their simplified interfaces. This is perfectly in line with the features required by our service, and we have therefore developed it to make it accessible even by patients who are not experienced with technology, through the use of standard procedures that they are already familiar with.

As for the activities reserved for the clinicians, we have taken a different approach. An additional section within the same application, designed to process requests and only available to the medical staff, could have been a viable option. However, we considered this to be impractical and instead chose to develop a dedicated system, accessible through a website, in which we sacrificed the ease of use in favor of a more comprehensive tool that could also be used on desktop computers.

These two pieces of software, although independent, still need to communicate with each other. To this end, we used the Firebase platform offered by Google, which provides an infrastructure for the development of mobile and web applications, comprising a number of services such as hosting, databases, patient authentication, and a simplified management of push and email notifications [21]. A sketch of the whole architecture is presented in Figure 1.

The development of smartphone applications is a process that normally follows two parallel paths, for Android and iOS devices, respectively. These two systems are fundamentally different from one another, and each has dedicated development tools. However, often developers do not need to use any platform-specific tool or feature, or even differentiate their products for the two operating systems. This holds true in our case as well, where speed of development was crucial to achieve the goal. For this reason, we opted for a hybrid development system that would allow simultaneous development on both operating systems. We chose React Native [22], an open-source framework made by Facebook to create mobile applications in JavaScript. Similarly, and for consistency, the dashboard was built using its counterpart for web applications, React [23].

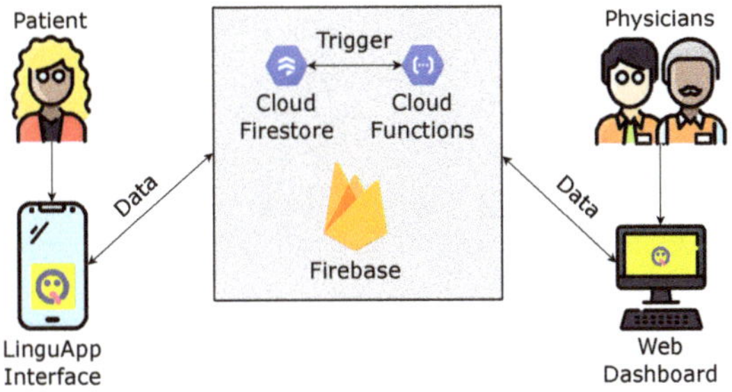

Figure 1. Simple sketch of the proposed methodology.

2.1. Decision Graph

The primary purpose of our application is to collect information about patients and their symptoms using a well-structured approach. This was accomplished by asking the patient to perform a self-inspection by choosing, from a set of fixed alternatives, the options that best fit their problem. We considered the possibility of allowing patients to openly describe their symptoms, but this could have led to inaccurate or incomplete information that would have required subsequent refinements. Instead, we wanted an exhaustive application in providing data and alternatives to the patient, starting from the first interaction. This observation led to the issue of properly structuring the progression between questions.

At first, we considered using a decision tree, but this turned out to be insufficiently flexible for our needs. This is because, in the considered survey, some of the questions are repeated in distinct paths and the use of a decision tree would result in unnecessary redundancies. Indeed, when using such a structure, a question may only be preceded by a specific series of answers, instead of several distinct series.

For this reason, we opted for an acyclic directed graph where each node represents a question, and, as such, contains a set of strings. In particular, each alternative is indicated by a string that can help in making a diagnosis (e.g., description of symptoms, presence of pre-existing conditions, lifestyle habits). Though not required, a node may also contain a header string that provides further details related to all alternatives. Each alternative is also associated with a reference to the next question, which can be interpreted as an edge in the graph (Figure 2). The keys of the JSON code, provided in English as Additional Material (see Appendix A), are the labels of the individual nodes. The first question, common to all subgraphs, is proposed to the patient and indicated here by the white circle; the small disks in gray represent the invitation to take photos. LinguApp notifies the specialists' team via email that a new request was added so that they can quickly assess the case and get in touch with the patient. Due to privacy reasons, no sensitive data is attached in the email.

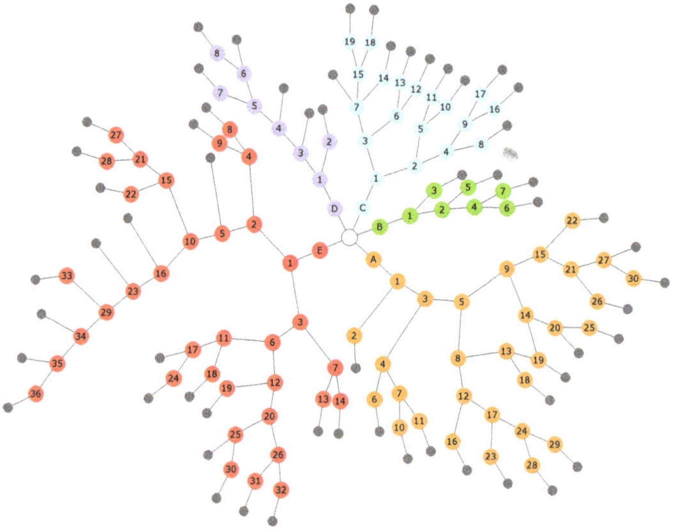

Figure 2. Graphical representation of the questionnaire. Colours indicate the five main branches, corresponding to the possible answers of the first query. Further details are provided in the Additional Material (Appendix A). The reader is referred to the electronic version of the article for interpretation of the colours in this figure.

Once we established the data structure, we needed to find a suitable way to represent and store it. We opted for the JSON format, as it is highly flexible and natively handled by both the JavaScript language and the Firebase's database service, called Firestore. Initially, one might think of nesting a node inside its ancestor, following the typical structure of a JSON file, but this is not adequate for our data structure, as, once again, it would describe a tree. The solution we have employed requires all nodes be stored at the same level and that each be associated with an identifying key. Our JSON representation can be examined in the Additional Material (Appendix A).

It is possible to represent the path that a patient follows through the graph by means of a list in which the keys of the visited nodes are stored. An algorithm for visualizing a path is implemented in both the mobile and web application and follows the pseudocode in Appendix A, Algorithm A1.

2.2. *Firebase Backend*

Firestore is the Firebase component that manages databases; it is structured in collections and each of them contains documents, which represent a set of key-value pairs. The most relevant collections for the functioning of our software are those that contain the surveys and the paths taken by the patients.

Each survey was mapped to a graph represented in JSON, as described in the previous section, and stored in a document within the same collection. The contents are maintained by system administrators, who have the option of adding new surveys and new questions in an existing one, though deletions cannot be made, as it would no longer be possible to interpret the paths previously taken by patients (i.e., we impose that our application is backward compatible).

The collection of paths contains one document for each path. The status for a path can be one of "draft", "awaiting photos", "awaiting feedback", and "completed". A path contains a reference to the patient who created it, the list of choices, an indication of the status and links to the associated photos, which are stored through the storage service. For security and privacy reasons, only administrators have access to the whole documents. When a patient completes the self-inspection, including uploading photos, members of the medical staff are notified via email, leveraging Firebase's cloud functions. Similarly, when clinicians provide feedback, the patient involved is notified via push notifications and email.

This service is available upon a sign-up procedure, which is structured in two steps. At first, an account is created through an authentication service (email, Google, Apple ID) and only afterwards do patients provide their personal data and a phone number that will be stored in a dedicated collection. The data entered is validated using other Firebase services.

Moreover, Firebase provides the Remote Config service, which allows administrators to quickly edit text and settings within the application without having to release an update on the stores: LinguApp will download new values at each startup, while the dashboard will update them every time the webpage is refreshed.

2.3. Mobile Application

When first launching LinguApp, the patient must sign up or log in using a previously created account. The first screen shows a short tutorial, after which the patient can start a new path or view a previously created one (Figure 3a).

During the creation of a new path, the patient is asked to select the survey category they consider most suitable among the available ones (Figure 3b). From this point on, the list of decisions made by the patient is treated as a stack that initially contains the key of the first node of the selected category. Any choice made by the patient results in its immediate synchronization on Firestore.

The screen that follows provides a dedicated interface for viewing and interacting with the decisions currently taken, allowing the patient to either advance by answering a new question, or go back to change a previously proposed answer (Figure 3c). The path is shown as a list, where each node corresponds to a panel. The list can be displayed in full or in a compact form: if an answer has yet to be provided, all of its alternatives are shown, whereas if an answer has already been given, it will be the only one displayed. This means that, by default, only one node at a time is fully displayed, namely the last one in the path. However, to allow patients to go back, we made it so that upon tapping a past question, its panel expands again. A question that is fully displayed allows interaction with its alternatives. Selecting one of them will truncate any following given answers and append the key of the node that is pointed to by the selected alternative. Further details on this procedure are provided in Appendix A, Algorithm A2.

When a patient reaches a terminal node, the path changes to "waiting for photos", and displays the interface for uploading photos. Upon successful submission, the status will change to "waiting for feedback". When a clinician provides feedback, it is shown on this screen. For the specific problem to solve, we preferred to make the patient shoot photos, but LinguApp can be modified to capture videos as well.

We have done our best to make the app as undemanding as possible in terms of operating system, hardware resources, and memory space. The minimum required version of Android is 4.1, released in 2012; the size to download the app from the store is about 23 megabytes, and after installation it takes about 46 megabytes. In the case of iOS, at least the 9.0 version is required, 24 megabytes have to be downloaded from the store, and just 16 megabytes are occupied on the device. These differences are due to the optimization policies of the respective operating systems.

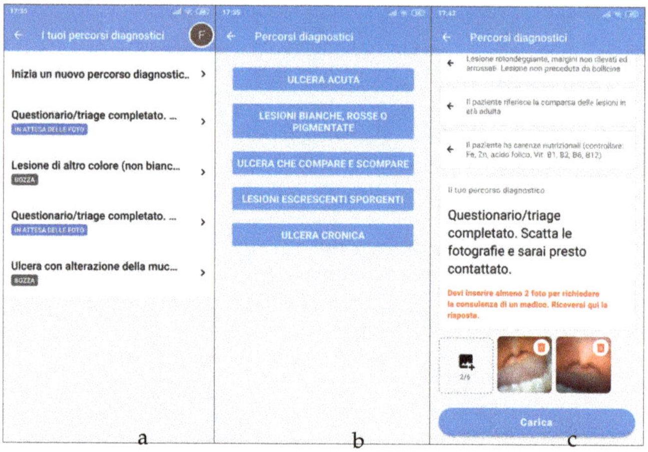

Figure 3. Requests started by a user with their relative statuses color-coded, e.g., "draft" in grey and "waiting for photos" in blue (**a**). First choice of a path (**b**). Request awaiting submission, with all choices already taken and showing the interface for adding photos (**c**). LinguApp features Italian phrases that can be translated quite easily (please see Additional Material).

2.4. Web Application

Login to the dashboard, which is run on Firebase's hosting service, is performed via email and password or via a Google account. The sign-up of clinicians is performed by the system administrators to prevent arbitrary individuals from accessing these functionalities. Although this procedure is cumbersome, developing a more extensive feature would be futile.

The web portal has a dedicated section for content management where it is possible to edit questions and answers. As already mentioned, the backward compatibility with previous completed paths limits clinicians' freedom of editing surveys. This is a minor limitation, though, as the surveys were designed to remain essentially unaltered.

The other, and most important, section is the one from which medical staff can review patient submissions. As all clinicians have equal access to this section, being able to distinguish between requests that still need attention and those that have already received feedback is essential for proper and effective cooperation. To achieve this, the completed requests are marked by a label. The details of a path are displayed in a dedicated page that shows the given answers, the photos included, and the patient's contact details. Once a clinician has formulated a feedback, based on the available information, the patient will be contacted via a dedicated input field on the page or through the contact information (Figure 4).

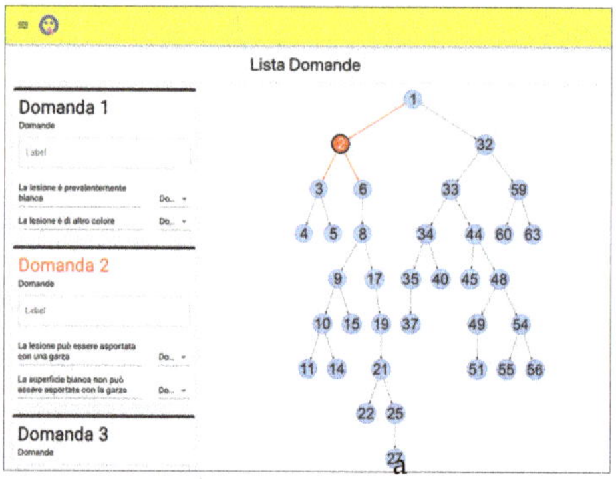

Figure 4. *Cont.*

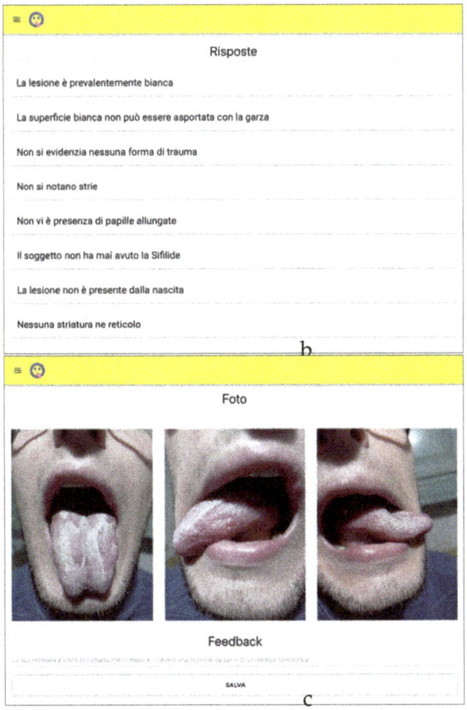

Figure 4. The web interface allows to create and modify the questionnaire, also through graphic representation (**a**). It is possible to delete or view details for an individual request on a dedicated page containing patient contact information, the selections made (**b**), and the attached photos (**c**). Sensitive data has been censored. LinguApp features Italian phrases that can be translated quite easily (please see Additional Material).

2.5. Privacy and Security

Confidentiality is fundamental in the medical field, so any application that operates in this area must provide strong guarantees on the treatment of user data. Patients that use LinguApp need to provide personal information such as their full name, email address, and phone number. To start a diagnostic path with a clinician, they also need to answer questions that could reveal more sensitive data, and then take pictures of their lesions. Our approach to preserving users' privacy and security is twofold.

First, we leverage the built-in security provided by all Firebase services, which is equivalent to that of mainstream products. Firebase rejects all requests coming from untrusted clients. Indeed, our clients have been configured for each of the three platforms, iOS, Android, and the web, through the use of private configuration files that guarantee their authority, and all communications are carried out through a private channel.

Second, we add a layer of protection by limiting the access to the resources, particularly to the collection of patients' data and paths and to their pictures. The access is controlled through a variety of Firebase services. First of all, the sign-up procedure makes use of Auth to ensure that all users, both patients and clinicians, have a personal account, and of Custom Claims to ensure that their account is "activated" before they can access any other functionality. In other words, users have to provide valid information, completing both steps of the sign-up process, before the service becomes available. When an "activated" user makes a request, only the user's own data will be disclosed. This is guaranteed via Security Rules that are applied in Firestore and Storage before a request is processed.

According to Firebase's best practices for security and privacy, these restrictions should be enough to ensure that the visibility of information is limited to the account, and by extension the patient, who created it. Indeed, even if a third party were to gain access to the clients' source code, they would not be able to obtain additional data due to server-side restrictions.

As noted in the Terms and Conditions of the software, all data collected via LinguApp can be accessed by clinicians at Department of Surgical Oncological and Stomatological Disciplines in Palermo, Italy, solely for diagnostic purposes and for health and administrative records required by law. If necessary, data might also be disclosed to a patient's treating clinician, other healthcare personnel, and dental laboratories. Additionally, in order to ensure European General Data Protection Regulation compliance, patients can download their data and request deletion, should they wish to do so.

3. Results and Discussion

LinguApp has made it possible, and still makes it possible, to manage patients who, for various reasons, require a prodromal remote consultation. On the basis of the anamnestic documentation provided online by the patients and the evaluation of the images sent, the medical team expresses its opinion on a therapeutic indication or on the need for further diagnostic investigations that require an in-person consultation. In this latter case, the appropriate hospital structure to manage the case is indicated [17,18]. During this pandemic period, the app has enabled numerous patients to find a solution to their problem without having to leave their homes. In other cases, the patient had to go to a hospital, but only after the medical team had recognized the real necessity, which is extremely important in order not to unnecessarily burden hospital facilities.

In this case, LinguApp has also enabled carrying out a remote triage which is essential in order to have access to health facilities in Italy, having assessed the low risk of COVID-19 positivity. The app has therefore made it possible to manage some patients at a remote distance but also to accept at the health facility low-risk patients with COVID-19 positivity, thus reducing the risk of patient mobility, which is essential for the containment of the pandemic infection itself. In particular, we believe it is useful to report, among the many requests for assistance, an emblematic case. It regards a disabled and bedridden patient. This consultation request was made by the relatives of the patient who had been experiencing serious difficulties in feeding for several days. From the anamnestic collection it was possible to highlight the frequent use of aerosol therapy containing corticosteroid drugs. The images highlighted the presence of numerous root residues, and the presence of oral extremely erythematous mucosae (Figure 5). Considering the reported semi-liquid diet, the medical team believed that the feeding difficulties could be caused by oral burning, probably related to drug-related mycotic overinfection and also related to the poor oral hygiene conditions due to the general health conditions of the patient. Therefore, it was recommended to follow a topical antifungal therapy for 15 days and also an improvement of oral hygiene conditions through the use of gauzes and a basifying agent based on water and bicarbonate. After 15 days, the patient reported the disappearance of any difficulty to eat and the reduction of the erythema of the oral mucosa.

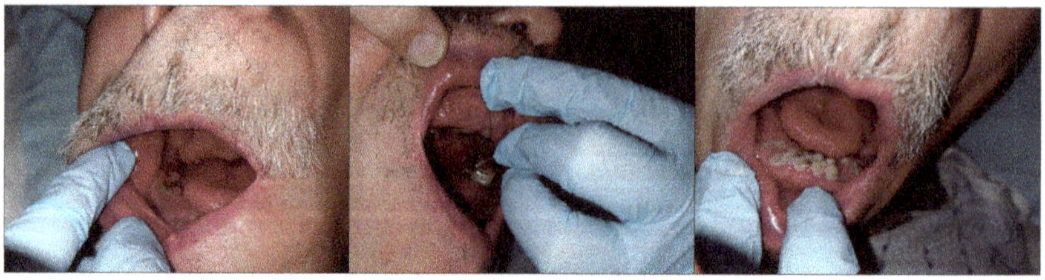

Figure 5. An anonymized real case study. Although no hospital examination was necessary, this example points out the effectiveness of the proposed methodology.

We think this case absolutely emblematic: indeed, the presence of the disabled patient in a hospital would have involved obvious difficulties, for example, his transport via dedicated means such as an ambulance. Moreover, it would have required the participation of several accompanying persons. The risk to which this patient would have been exposed with numerous comorbidities in case of COVID-19 infection would have placed his life in serious danger, as well as his family members.

4. Conclusions

The search for pathological formations or dysembryogenic alterations that can affect the soft tissues of the mouth, either as the only organ in which they are found, or as expression of pathologies that also occur in other sites, shows how many lesions clinically resemble each other [17–20]. The similarity among the appearance of many lesions represents a difficulty to be overcome to allow the clinician to arrive at a definitive diagnosis. It has been considered the existence both of common characteristics among some pathologies and the presence of univocal characteristics. The combination of all these features allowed us to give a presumptive name to the observed pathology, as every pathology will always have univocal features, but often they are not immediately detectable. We believe that our methodology can help to follow a method that includes, unknowingly, the differential diagnosis [19,20].

We underline that the algorithm has been realized using the clinical and histological features reported in specialized articles and books, but we do not exclude that in some subjects, the pathology may present a different clinical picture or that the patient may report information that is not completely accurate. In this case, the use of LinguApp could lead to an incorrect diagnosis; however, we believe that, for many patients, following this type of pathway can lead to a correct diagnosis in a quick and easy way. Therefore, we consider fundamental a meticulous anamnesis of the patient, in order to have detailed information on the evolution of the lesion, on the symptomatology of the same, and on the habits/risk factors of the patient, in order to be able to answer in an unequivocal way the questions posed in the algorithm [17,19].

Moreover, the use of the application over time will refine the type of questions, making them increasingly targeted. However, there is no doubt that the idea of being able to create sets of diseases and, within these, gradually find differences and then create subgroups, may be one of the correct methods to reach the recognition of the disease and then the diagnosis.

The proposed methodology is still in use today and provides a fast track to hospital admission for patients requiring direct intervention, without the need to have contact with any further people at risk of COVID-19 infection. This best practice could continue to be pursued after the contingent emergency as it generally simplifies the procedure from both the healthcare personnel and patient perspectives and it shortens the waiting time.

Finally, we point out that our application has been developed in flexible and logically separated modules. This would allow to quickly modify each single module to deal with different diagnostic problems, based on a proper questionnaire and on the submission of photos or videos. For example, LinguApp can be addressed to general practitioners, dentists, pediatricians, and dermatologists, presenting a more specific questionnaire for the collaboration of the various branch specialists. This is a strong point compared to other similar mobile applications currently available, specific to particular diseases.

So far, apps have been developed in various countries to track infected people (generally, on a voluntary basis) [24–28] or to make diagnoses through established approaches [29–33] or neural network-based techniques [34] that require extensive hardware resources. The Italian government has recently confirmed the sponsorship of remote diagnostics in all forms. Obviously, preference should be given to user-friendly tools that do not require special assets from the medical staff and especially from patients. From a general point of view, mobile technologies cannot replace a direct contact with the patient, but can contribute to the rapid diagnosis and maintain a high safety level for both operators and patients themselves, limiting their access to specialist facilities only in cases that are really necessary.

Author Contributions: Conceptualization, G.A.S., P.M. and C.L.; methodology, M.F., C.L., G.M., A.T. and F.T.; software, M.F., G.M., A.T. and F.T.; validation, A.M.; formal analysis, P.M., G.A.S. and C.V.; investigation, M.F., C.L., G.M., P.M., G.A.S., A.T., F.T. and C.V.; data curation, G.M., P.M. and C.V.; writing—original draft preparation, P.M., G.A.S. and C.V.; writing—review and editing, A.M. P.M., G.A.S. and C.V.; supervision, G.A.S. and C.V. All authors have read and agreed to the published version of the manuscript.

Funding: This research received no external funding.

Institutional Review Board Statement: All procedures performed in this studies involving human participants were in accordance with the ethical standards of the institutional and/or national research committee and with the 1964 Helsinki declaration and its later amendments or comparable ethical standards.

Informed Consent Statement: Informed consent was obtained from all subjects involved in the study.

Conflicts of Interest: The authors declare no conflict of interest.

Appendix A

The questionnaire in JSON format currently used by LinguApp is provided as Additional Material together with a short video to show how the Web and Mobile interfaces work. All these files can be downloaded at https://tinyurl.com/linguapp, accessed on 10 January 2022.

We introduce here a couple of main snippets. This codes refer to the actual questions that are proposed according to Figure 2.

When a path needs to be rendered, it is passed as state to Algorithm A1, which reads the key of each node in the list. Using this key, we can access the node's label, if one is available, and the text of all its questions. A variant of this code is used to display, for all but the last node, only the selected alternative, instead of all of them.

Algorithm A1 Current decision display.

```
input: list state containing the current decisions
for i ← 1 to size(state) do
    key ← state[i]
    if hasLabel(key) then
        text ← getLabel(key)
        displayLabel(text)
    end
    questions ← getQuestions(key)
    for j ← 1 to size(questions) do
        text ← getQuestionText(questions[j])
        displayQuestion(text)
    end
end
```

Algorithm A2 is executed when an alternative is selected, passing the index of the node involved in the stack as current and the index of the chosen alternative from the questions array as answer. This procedure removes the nodes in the path that come after current, which are only present if the patient is going back, and then adds the key of the node that is pointed to by the selected alternative.

Algorithm A2 Decision stack update.

```
input: index of the current active question, index of the new answer
while current < size(state) do
    pop(state)
end
key ← peek(state)
questions ← getQuestions(key)
nextQuestion ← questions[answer]
push(state, nextQuestion)
```

References

1. Estai, M.; Kanagasingam, Y.; Xiao, D.; Vignarajan, J.; Bunt, S.; Kruger, E.; Tennant, M. End-user acceptance of a cloud-based teledentistry system and Android phone app for remote screening for oral diseases. *J. Telemed. Telecare* **2017**, *23*, 44–52. [CrossRef] [PubMed]
2. Meagher, R.; Kousvelari, E. Mobile oral heath technologies based on saliva. *Oral Dis.* **2018**, *24*, 194–197. [CrossRef] [PubMed]
3. Motta, A.; Rodrigues, K. Could we benefit from oral self-examination during the COVID-19 pandemic? *Oral Oncol.* **2020**, *107*, 104840. [CrossRef] [PubMed]
4. Zhang, C.; Fan, L.; Chai, Z.; Yu, C.; Song, J. Smartphone and medical application use among dentists in china. *BMC Med. Inform. Decis. Mak.* **2020**, *20*, 213. [CrossRef]
5. Acharya, P.; Mathur, M. Smartphone applications for the triage of skin lesions using machine learning: Time to integrate the clinical information? *J. Eur. Acad. Dermatol. Venereol.* **2020**, *34*, e424–e425. [CrossRef]
6. Jheng, Y.-C.; Chou, Y.-B.; Kao, C.-L.; Yarmishyn, A.; Hsu, C.-C.; Lin, T.-C.; Chen, P.-Y.; Kao, Z.-K.; Chen, S.-J.; Hwang, D.-K. A novelty route for smartphone-based artificial intelligence approach to ophthalmic screening. *J. Chin. Med. Assoc.* **2020**, *83*, 898–899. [CrossRef]
7. de Haan, K.; Koydemir, H.; Rivenson, Y.; Tseng, D.; Dyne, E.V.; Bakic, L.; Karinca, D.; Liang, K.; Ilango, M.; Gumustekin, E.; et al. Automated screening of sickle cells using a smartphone-based microscope and deep learning. *NPJ Digit. Med.* **2020**, *3*, 76. [CrossRef]
8. Byrne, S.; Kotze, B.; Ramos, F.; Casties, A.; Harris, A. Using a mobile health device to manage severe mental illness in the community: What is the potential and what are the challenges? *Aust. N. Z. J. Psychiatry* **2020**, *54*, 964–969. [CrossRef]
9. Gaydina, T.; Dvornikova, E. Efficacy of smartphone-compatible optical instrument for assessing melanocytic nevi for malignancy. *Bull. Russ. State Med. Univ.* **2020**, *5*, 108–112.
10. Yu, H.; Yang, F.; Rajaraman, S.; Ersoy, I.; Moallem, G.; Poostchi, M.; Palaniappan, K.; Antani, S.; Maude, R.; Jaeger, S. Malaria Screener: A smartphone application for automated malaria screening. *BMC Infect. Dis.* **2020**, *20*, 825. [CrossRef]
11. Kumar, H.; Tanveer, N.; Dixit, S.; Diwan, H.; Naz, F. Smartphone-assisted tele-gynepathology: A pilot study. *Obstet. Gynaecol. Res.* **2020**, *46*, 1879–1884. [CrossRef]
12. Lorca-Cabrera, J.; Marti-Arques, R.; Albacar-Rioboo, N.; Raigal-Aran, L.; Roldan-Merino, J.; Ferre-Grau, C. Mobile applications for caregivers of individuals with chronic conditions and/or diseases: Quantitative content analysis. *Int. J. Med. Inform.* **2021**, *145*, e104310. [CrossRef]
13. Singhal, S.; Mohapatra, S.; Quinone, C. Reviewing Teledentistry Usage in Canada during COVID-19 to Determine Possible Future Opportunities. *Int. J. Environ. Res. Public Health* **2020**, *19*, 31. [CrossRef]
14. Maspero, C.; Abate, A.; Cavagnetto, D.; Morsi, M.E.; Fama, A.; Farronato, M. Available Technologies, Applications and Benefits of Teleorthodontics. A Literature Review and Possible Applications during the COVID-19 Pandemic. *J. Clin. Med.* **2020**, *9*, 1891. [CrossRef]
15. Matarese, M.; Cervino, G.; Fiorillo, L.; Stelitano, C.; Bellantoni, M.I.; Meto, A.; Lucchina, A.G.; Tornello, F.; Anastasi, M.R.; Rengo, C. A cohort study on anticoagulant therapy risks in dental patients after multiple extractions. *Minerva Dent. Oral Sci.* **2021**, *70*, 196–205. [CrossRef]
16. Fiorillo, L.; Cervino, G.; Matarese, M.; D'Amico, C.; Surace, G.; Paduano, V.; Fiorillo, M.T.; Moschella, A.; Bruna, A.L.; Romano, G.L.; et al. COVID-19 Surface Persistence—A Recent Data Summary and Its Importance for Medical and Dental Settings. *Int. J. Environ. Res. Public Health* **2020**, *17*, 3132. [CrossRef]
17. Scardina, G.; Pisano, T.; Messina, P. Oral mucositis. review of literature. *N. Y. State Dent. J.* **2010**, *76*, 34–38.
18. Scardina, G.; Carini, F.; Maresi, E.; Valenza, V.; Messina, P. Evaluation of the clinical and histological effectiveness of isotretinoin in the therapy of oral leukoplakia—Ten years of experience: Is management still up to date and effective? *Methods Find Exp. Clin. Pharmacol.* **2006**, *28*, 115–119. [CrossRef]
19. Scardina, G.; Ruggieri, A.; Messina, P.; Maresi, E. Angiogenesis of oral lichen planus: A possible pathogenetic mechanism. *Med. Oral Patol. Oral Cir. Bucal* **2009**, *14*, e558–e562. [CrossRef]
20. Scardina, G.; Ruggieri, A.; Maresi, E.; Messina, P. Angiogenesis in oral lichen planus: An in vivo and immunohistological evaluation. *Arch. Immunol. Ther. Exp.* **2011**, *59*, 457–462. [CrossRef]

21. Firebase. Available online: https://firebase.google.com (accessed on 10 January 2022).
22. React Native. Available online: https://reactnative.dev (accessed on 10 January 2022).
23. React. Available online: https://reactjs.org (accessed on 10 January 2022).
24. Immuni. Available online: www.immuni.italia.it (accessed on 10 January 2022).
25. RadarCovid. Available online: https://radarcovid.gob.es (accessed on 10 January 2022).
26. NHS COVID-19. Available online: https://covid19.nhs.uk (accessed on 10 January 2022).
27. COVID Alert. Available online: www.canada.ca/covid-alert (accessed on 10 January 2022).
28. TousAntiCovid. Available online: https://bonjour.tousanticovid.gouv.fr (accessed on 10 January 2022).
29. Coelho, R.; Gesù, V.D.; Bosco, G.L.; Tanaka, J.; Valenti, C. Shape-based features for cat ganglion retinal cells classification. *Real-Time Imaging* **2002**, *8*, 213–226. [CrossRef]
30. Bellavia, F.; Cacioppo, A.; Lupaşcu, C.; Messina, P.; Scardina, G.; Tegolo, D.; Valenti, C. A non-parametric segmentation methodology for oral videocapillaroscopic images. *Comput. Methods Programs Biomed.* **2014**, *114*, 240–246. [CrossRef]
31. Sciortino, G.; Tegolo, D.; Valenti, C. Automatic detection and measurement of nuchal translucency. *Comput. Biol. Med.* **2017**, *82*, 12–20. [CrossRef]
32. Giudice, A.; Barone, S.; Muraca, D.; Averta, F.; Diodati, F.; Antonelli, A.; Fortunato, L. Can teledentistry improve the monitoring of patients during the Covid-19 dissemination? A descriptive pilot study. *Int. J. Environ. Res. Public Health* **2020**, *17*, 10. [CrossRef]
33. Tobias, G.; Spanier, A. Developing a mobile app (iGAM) to promote gingival health by professional monitoring of dental selfies: User-centered design approach. *Int. J. Environ. Res. Public Health* **2020**, *8*, 8. [CrossRef]
34. Khanagar, S.B.; Al-Ehaideb, A.; Maganur, P.C.; Vishwanathaiah, S.; Patil, S.; Baeshen, H.A.; Sarode, S.C.; Bhandi, S. Developments, application, and performance of artificial intelligence in dentistry. *J. Dent. Sci.* **2021**, *16*, 508–522. [CrossRef]

International Journal of
Environmental Research and Public Health

MDPI

Review

The Impact of the COVID-19 Pandemic on Dentistry and Dental Education: A Narrative Review

Ancuta Goriuc [1,†], Darius Sandu [2,†], Monica Tatarciuc [3,*] and Ionut Luchian [4]

1 Department of Biochemistry, Faculty of Dental Medicine, "Grigore T. Popa" University of Medicine and Pharmacy, 700115 Iasi, Romania; ancuta.goriuc@umfiasi.ro
2 Faculty of Dental Medicine, "Grigore T. Popa" University of Medicine and Pharmacy, 16 Universitatii St., 700115 Iasi, Romania; darius-valentin.lr.sandu@students.umfiasi.ro
3 Department of Dental Technology, Faculty of Dental Medicine, "Grigore T. Popa" University of Medicine and Pharmacy, 700115 Iasi, Romania
4 Department of Periodontology, Faculty of Dental Medicine, "Grigore T. Popa" University of Medicine and Pharmacy, 700115 Iasi, Romania; ionut.luchian@umfiasi.ro
* Correspondence: monica.tatarciuc@umfiasi.ro; Tel.: +40-726-687-830
† These authors contributed equally to this work.

Abstract: Dentists and dental staff have an increased risk of airborne infection with pathogens such as SARS-CoV-2 since they are exposed to high levels of droplets and aerosols produced during specific dental procedures. Hence, new guidelines such as patient screening and temperature control, air purification, space, surface and hand sanitizing and the use of protective equipment and physical barriers have been successfully implemented. In addition, the use of teledentistry has expanded considerably in pediatric dentistry, orthodontics, oral medicine and periodontics in order to address oral and dental health issues during the COVID-19 pandemic while minimizing virus transmission. Thus, teleconsultation, telediagnosis, teletriage, teletreatment and telemonitoring have emerged as valuable tools not only in the delivery of care, but also in the academic and research training of dental health professionals. This narrative review summarizes the current literature on the impact of the pandemic on dental care, dental staff and dental education, with an emphasis on how newly emerging protocols and technologies can be successfully utilized as integral parts of various branches of the dental practice and their future implications without compromising patient care.

Keywords: SARS-CoV-2 infection; dental healthcare; dental training; teledentistry; pandemic; dental aerosols

Citation: Goriuc, A.; Sandu, D.; Tatarciuc, M.; Luchian, I. The Impact of the COVID-19 Pandemic on Dentistry and Dental Education: A Narrative Review. *Int. J. Environ. Res. Public Health* **2022**, *19*, 2537. https://doi.org/10.3390/ijerph19052537

Academic Editors: Giuseppe Alessandro Scardina and Jimmy Efird

Received: 10 December 2021
Accepted: 30 January 2022
Published: 22 February 2022

Publisher's Note: MDPI stays neutral with regard to jurisdictional claims in published maps and institutional affiliations.

1. Introduction

According to data provided by the World Health Organization (WHO), the new coronavirus, SARS-CoV-2, had caused 5,493,846 deaths globally by 10 January 2022, of which approximately 20% were recorded in the USA. Multiple factors are responsible for differences in contamination and mortality due to SARS-CoV-2 between countries. These include the implementation of domestic policies to control the spread of infection, vaccination, population density, comorbidities and the proportion of the ageing population, to name a few [1]. This has led to a significant variation in the degree of infectiveness and mortality (Tables 1 and 2) [2].

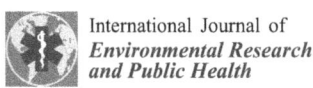

Among medical practitioners, dentists and dental staff have an increased risk of being infected with airborne pathogens such as SARS-CoV-2 because they are always exposed to droplets and aerosols produced during specific treatment procedures. Transmission may occur due to the inhalation of droplets and aerosols from an infected individual or by direct contact with mucous membranes, oral fluids and contaminated instruments or surfaces. To evaluate the effects of intraoral and extraoral aspiration on the spread of infection during dental treatments, the bacterial colonization of droplets and aerosols was evaluated following simulations of scaling by the dentist and dental hygienist in three healthy volunteers. Extraoral aspiration has been shown to reduce the production of droplets and aerosols, and since it is restricted to the left and back of the dental chair, right-handed operators could perform treatment with relatively low contact with the pathogens. This study suggests that both aspiration methods were effective; however, extraoral aspiration was more effective in reducing the number of droplets and aerosols compared to intraoral aspiration or a lack of aspiration [3]. Furthermore, it has been shown that saliva represents a potential source of contamination for many patients. This aspect is of critical importance in public health management, not only for SARS-CoV-2, but also for other pathogens, considering the high rate of exposure to saliva by dental professionals [4].

Table 1. SARS-CoV-2 infection rate by August 2021 [2].

SARS-CoV-2	Percentage
United States	18.19%
India	15.22%
Brazil	9.65%
Russia	3.17%
France	3.11%
United Kingdom	3.06%
Spain	2.25%
Romania	6.87%
Average	7.69%

Table 2. SARS-CoV-2 cases and mortality rate by 10 January 2022 (https://coronavirus.jhu.edu/data/mortality (accessed on 26 August 2021)).

Country	Cases Confirmed	Deaths	Case Fatality (%)
Peru	2,358,685	203,019	8.6%
Brazil	22,529,183	620,251	2.8%
Belgium	2,231,686	28,459	1.3%
Italy	7,436,939	139,038	1.9%
Mexico	4,125,388	300,334	7.3%
United States	60,074,429	837,594	1.4%
United Kingdom	14,563,769	150,634	1.0%
Ecuador	559,950	33,699	6.0%
Romania	1,844,537	59,011	3.2%
Spain	7,164,906	89,934	1.3%
Portugal	1,499,976	19,029	1.3%
France	12,218,022	126,427	1.0%
South Africa	3,526,054	92,453	2.6%
Iran	6,206,405	131,878	2.1%
Russia	10,470,006	309,787	3.0%
Greece	1,507,616	21,394	1,4%
Austria	1,339,421	13,848	1.0%
Germany	7,553,743	114,033	1.5%
Average	970,464,876	163,519,323	2.70%

Since COVID-19 is primarily spread through droplets and aerosols, it could reasonably be assumed that dentistry might be among the professions with the highest mortality rate [1]. However, when the number of deaths was examined in England and Wales between March and December 2020, there was no evidence of a higher mortality rate among dentists caused by COVID-19. This led to the conclusion that the low infection rate of dentists might be due to the rigorous safety protocols implemented. The American Dental Association (ADA), as well as most European dental organizations, recommends patient prescreening before visiting the clinic, allowing only one patient at a time in the waiting room, measuring staff and patients' temperatures, hand washing and sanitizing, access to sanitizers for patients, disinfection of surfaces, personal protection equipment for the medical team, disposable shoe covers for patients, use of UV lamps and other air purifiers and high-efficiency aspiration during treatments (Figure 1) [1,5]. For example, Butera et al. suggested the use of the bio-inspired systems in nonsurgical periodontal treatment in order to reduce the risk of bacteremia and aerosol generation and improve clinical, microbiological and immunological parameters by decreasing bacterial load [6].

This qualitative, narrative review summarizes the most recent literature on the effects of the COVID-19 pandemic on dental practice and dental education, as well as the use of teledentistry in the delivery of oral and dental care to avoid virus contamination. Research and review papers were identified and selected using Scopus, PubMed and Web of Science scientific databases. Commentaries, letters and in vitro studies were excluded from the analysis. The paper describes in a comprehensive and critical manner, the effects of COVID-19 pandemic on the delivery of oral and dental care and dental education and its impact on current and future dental practice.

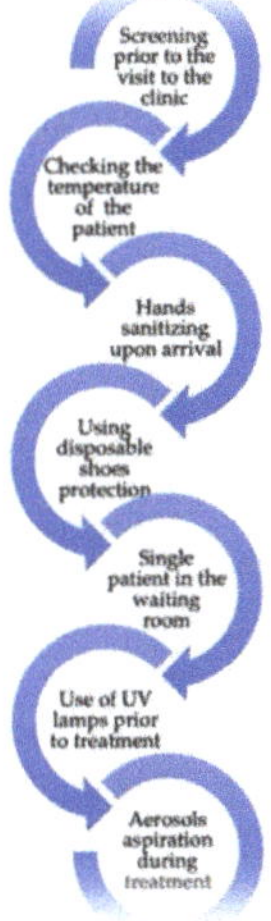

Figure 1. Safety protocol for dental patients during the COVID-19 pandemic.

2. COVID-19 and the New Approach to Dental Healthcare

Teledentistry has been defined as "the remote practice of dentistry by oral health professionals, within the limits of their practices, via the use of information and communication technology" [6]. Its objectives should not depart from those of in-person care, and may include diagnosis, prevention and post-treatment monitoring, specialist advice, treatment, prescription, referrals and other practices. Approximately 80% of dentists have adopted precautionary recommendations and modified them according to the type and particularities of each dental treatment [7]. For example, to increase the safety of the working team, a recent study showed that approximately 30% of dentists wore additional protective equipment, applied sanitation and ventilation procedures beyond those recommended by the guidelines and local health authorities, preferred to treat infected patients or those suspected of infection at the end of the working day and used an FFP3 mask during treatment. Approximately 78% of dentists replaced the FFP2 mask after eight hours of use, even when treating non-contaminated patients, and 62% covered the FFP2 mask with an FFP1 surgical mask [7].

Furthermore, 89% of dentists recommended oral rinses with solutions based on hydrogen peroxide and chlorhexidine before commencing therapeutic procedures. The combination of hydrogen peroxide with chlorhexidine solutions has been shown in vitro to be more effective than either solution alone in preventing transmission of SARS-CoV-2 [7]. Other studies have shown a decrease in salivary viral load after a 30 s mouth and oropharynx gargle with 15 mL of 1.5% or 3% hydrogen peroxide solution or 0.12% chlorhexidine solution [8]. Likewise, brief (30 s) rinses with 0.2%, 0.4% or 0.5% povidone–iodine (9 mL) or 0.05% cetylpyridinium chloride (15 mL) have been proven to be effective. Similar effects were obtained with cetrimide rinses in oncologic patients. However, the degree to which these solutions are effective in preventing or decreasing SARS-CoV-2 contamination risks, particularly in vulnerable populations, still need to be examined [9].

Although SARS-CoV-2 has a predominantly airborne transmission, salivary contamination can be controlled much easier in dental offices. For example, recent studies that examined increasing suction capacity by using a large volume of air (150 mm Hg or 325 L/min) suggest that this measure may be sufficient to eliminate viral contamination [7]. To further increase safety at work, Italian dentists have adopted, as a preventative measure, ventilation of dental treatment rooms after examination of each patient, regardless of the dental treatment performed. In rooms with poor mechanical ventilation, portable air filters with a high-efficiency particulate air filter (HEPA) have effectively reduced aerosol accumulation and accelerated aerosol removal [10]. Taken together, these studies show that new measures put in place in dental offices significantly mitigate the risks of SARS-CoV-2 contamination, and the risk of contracting COVID-19 in the dental office is relatively low [11].

3. Dental Public Health Issues during the COVID-19 Pandemic

A recent study conducted in Italy showed a state of normalcy in dental practices after the initial wave of COVID-19 pandemic. Since its onset, Italian dentists have experienced high levels of anxiety and stress, mainly due to the rapid spread of SARS-CoV-2 at the national level and the need for rapid adaptation to the new health standards in dental offices [7]. Approximately 80% of Italian dentists resumed their regular activity after the first quarantine. However, there were some geographical differences due to the evolution of the virus over time. For example, the reopening rate of dental offices ranged from 36% in the United Kingdom to 47% in Palestine, while in Italy and the USA this figure reached 99%. Approximately 80% of dentists have adopted preventative measures and adapted them to specific dental treatments [7]. Notwithstanding these changes, dental offices incurred significant financial losses of over 70% due to the COVID-19 pandemic. In a survey conducted by the British Dental Association, 70% of dental clinics reported that they could only remain viable and maintain their usual number of employees for up to three months [7].

4. Pre-, during and Post-Pandemic Particular Aspects of Dental Treatments

A recent study highlighted the changes in the spectrum of procedures performed before and during the pandemic. For example, during the COVID-19 pandemic, the number of conservative procedures, such as coronal restorations or root canal fillings, decreased significantly, while the percentage of surgical procedures increased significantly. In the following months, the decrease in the number of patients was offset by an increased number of procedures per visit [12,13]. Likewise, several changes were recommended when performing various treatment procedures. For example, the mechanochemical treatment of carious lesions was carried out using hand tools instead of rotary ones. Similarly, for periodontal treatments, manual scaling was chosen over ultrasonic scaling. In cases of symptomatic irreversible pulpitis, biological methods, such as pulpotomy or pulpectomy, were recommended as much as possible [14]. On the other hand, in patients with extensive destruction of the hard dental tissue accompanied by severe pain, it was necessary to opt for the extraction of the affected tooth. Thus, it was possible to reduce the risk of infection, shorten treatment time and minimize repeated visits. In the case of excessive bleeding, multiple extractions or other oral surgeries, resorbable sutures were preferred. Specific interventions have been performed in pediatric patients to reduce aerosol-generating procedures and use non-invasive or minimally invasive methods. For example, fissure sealing, the topical application of varnishes and resin infiltration using the ICON method, were chosen in order to stop the evolution of non-cavitary carious lesions. At the same time, to minimize virus transmission and contamination, there was an increase in the number of certain procedures, such as indirect capping, atraumatic restorative treatment, provisional therapeutic restorations, the Hall technique and the application of diamine silver fluoride [13].

5. Teledentistry and COVID-19

Telemedicine has proven to be an effective tool in mitigating some of the effects caused by the imposition of restrictive measures during the COVID-19 pandemic. Several authors have suggested that the lack of coherence in the implementation of telemedicine as a solution for continuous medical education is one reason for the absence of uniform protocols for aerosol-generating procedures [14]. For example, dentists in the UK changed the way they approached clinical cases and developed a triage system using remote consultations. The treatment was limited to advice, analgesia and first-line antimicrobial therapy, with the goal of reducing the risk of transmission. COVID-19-positive patients, confirmed by RT-PCR, were directed to in-person treatment only in emergency dental centers, which have been previously authorized for this purpose [1].

Teledentistry has been increasingly used by dental schools during the pandemic. Although there are regional differences in isolation policies, the severity of the outbreak and the availability of resources have greatly impacted the functioning of dental schools during the pandemic, although the responses of dental institutions to the COVID-19 pandemic show some similarities. For example, distance learning was the only alternative to theoretical dental education in many institutions. While e-learning already existed, it evolved and expanded as a result of the COVID-19 pandemic, with the use of synchronous online teaching methods when interacting with participants [15]. In Italy, for example, telemedicine played a key role in reducing the spread of COVID-19 from the start of the pandemic. A number of teledentistry platforms such as OloHealth® have emerged since 2019 and are dedicated to the prevention and management of oral malignant disorders in addition to improvement of oral health, in order to reduce unnecessary travel and loss of productivity [16]. Likewise, teledentistry has been used successfully when treating patients with more complex oral pathologies by carrying out photographic teleconsultations for the first visits and for subsequent evaluations, thus ensuring a good remote patient management (Figure 2). After an adequate anamnesis by videocall and photographic evaluations during the first visit, patients were followed up with remote evaluations of their pathologies, such as fungal infections, dry mouth syndrome, sialolithiasis, traumatic ulcers, third molar pericoronitis and others [17].

Telemedicine was further used in cases that would normally require clinical examination in order to distinguish between potentially malignant lesions from those that were truly malignant and necessitated immediate attention. This allowed dentists to keep patients with precancerous lesions, osteonecrosis of the jaw associated with medication and autoimmune diseases under control by comparing recently received photos with the last photos taken at the dental clinic. For these pathologies, clinical changes were evaluated to determine the risk of malignant processes and manage possible recurrences, infections, pain and stability of lesions [16]. For example, Machado et al. emphasized the importance of oral telediagnosis when examining a 49-year-old female patient with controlled diabetes and symptomatic pinkish nodular lesions affecting the buccal mucosa, associated with purple spots on the skin. The dentist took photos with a short description using the WhatsApp platform and recommended a hematological examination based on idiopathic purpura. Severe thrombocytopenia was confirmed, and the patient was referred to the hospital for specialized systemic treatment with steroid medication [18]. When teledentistry is not available or cannot be used, saliva tests can be employed as a solution for screening patients with minimal physical contact given the strong link between salivary diagnosis and oncologic pathology [19].

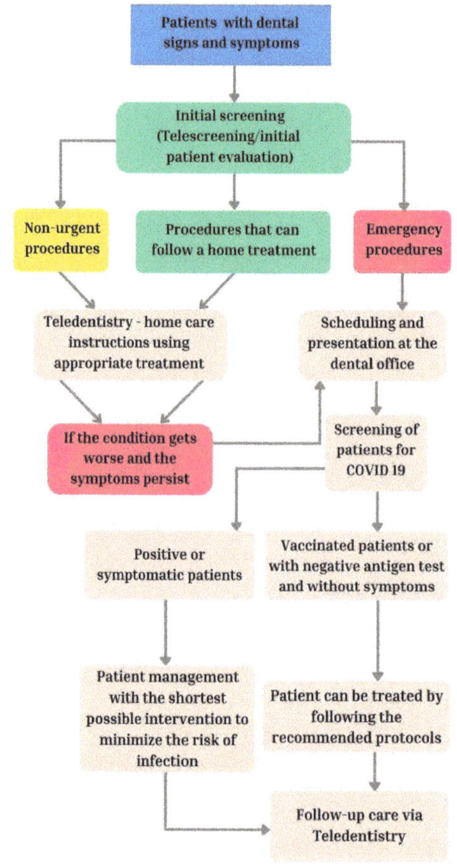

Figure 2. Management of dental protocols during COVID-19 pandemic.

Notwithstanding, teledentistry appears to be a promising tool in the remote management of patients requiring non-surgical or surgical treatment, especially by reducing costs and waiting times [15]. To this end, patients that need regular treatment for chronic conditions, geriatric patients or those with special needs, and patients living in remote, less-accessible areas can benefit the most from teledentistry. This can lead to reduction in the number of visits to the dental office, shorter waiting times, decreased no-show appointments, and reduced unnecessary exposure of healthy patients. The efficacy of teledentistry has mostly been studied in pediatric dentistry, oral medicine, orthodontics and periodontics for several procedures and with various degrees of success. For teledentistry to be effective, it requires an educated patient not only familiar with the new digital technologies (i.e., taking high-quality intraoral digital images, data storage, virtual communications using various apps, etc.) but also with basic dental knowledge [20]. For example, knowledge of the management of orthodontic appliances or teeth eruption, which represent a significant portion of emergency visits, can reduce office visits by approximately 20 percent. Fixing a loose or poking orthodontic wire or appliance, smaller fractures or tissue trauma can all be handled by teledentistry and avoid in-person visits. Indeed, some studies have shown that nearly half of all dental emergencies can be managed utilizing teledentistry. However, some of these procedures such as chronic pain, dental caries, severe trauma, fractures and orthodontic treatments would need to be evaluated frequently to avoid unnecessary delays that may lead to later complications such as infections. Not all dental practices and specialties are prepared or have the expertise for successful use of teledentistry, and it requires significant resources and infrastructure. For this reason, there is a wide range of teledentistry applications and its use varies across countries, regions, dental specialties and offices. Irrespective of these differences, the most important advantage lies in triaging patients, reducing the number of site visits and, in doing so, reducing exposure to pathogens such as SARS-CoV-2 [21].

In addition to the various devices that can be used in telemedicine, instant messaging applications have become increasingly popular for better communication between doctor and the patient. For example, WhatsApp-based teleradiology consultation proved to be an effective tool for interpreting X-rays with different dental pathologies [22]. Furthermore, dental telemedicine can be successfully applied during the follow-up of patients who have undergone oral and maxillofacial surgery, although more work is required to determine patients' compliance and doctors' attitudes towards integrating remote dentistry in the standard protocols of telemedicine [23].

6. The Impact of COVID-19 on Dental Staff

It is well established that COVID-19 had a significant impact on nurses working in the field of dentistry, which affected the quality of medical services. Chronic diseases, immunodeficiencies, the risk of SARS-CoV-2 infection, working in a private environment and family responsibilities associated with financial risks caused by the pandemic have all contributed to significant increases in anxiety, burn-outs and other mental health disorders [24]. This necessitates collective actions at the government level and a set of measures that can contribute both to the prevention and treatment of these manifestations [24,25]. Among dental staff, dental hygienists have been greatly impacted by the pandemic given the high risk of occupational contamination via aerosol loading due to their work in the maintenance of periodontal health and prevention of dental diseases. Although there are differences in the application of working protocols of prophylaxis, for assistants working in the private sector compared to those working in the public health system [24], the emphasis has been on minimizing the use of aerosol-generating procedures [25]. The existence of protective equipment for dental teams, an adequate infrastructure as well as the correct management of patients, all contributed to an increase in trust and safety within medical teams [24]. For example, a recent study conducted in the Czech Republic showed that well-chosen anti-epidemic measures adopted by dental professionals can reduce occupational infection risks associated with SARS-CoV-2 [26]. On the other hand, other studies examining the knowledge, attitudes and practices of the Turkish pediatric dentists, showed a satisfactory level of knowledge regarding COVID-19 prevention, although infection control measures could have been better implemented [27].

7. The Impact of COVID-19 on Dental Academic Environments

7.1. Emotional and Psychological Effects

Academics working in the field of dentistry have been subjected to a high level of stress during the COVID-19 pandemic, not only related to teaching and research activities but also to concerns related to the possibility of contaminating their family members [28]. This triggered an immediate and acute need for developing and implementing psychological support measures to reduce the level of mental stress among members of the academic staff. For example, Balkaran et al. recommended the use of meditation, specialized counselling and holding seminars for health promotion as therapeutic measures [28]. Similarly, a plethora of measures have been proposed for dental students, given the critical role of mental health in the educational evolution and behavioral development of dental students preparing for medical careers [29,30]. Chronic cardiovascular diseases, smoking and being female, as well as the economic impact of SARS-CoV-2 on the dental profession, have been shown to negatively affect the psychological status of dental students [24].

The COVID-19 pandemic has led to an increase in negative emotional states among students. Students were the population group most affected by the pandemic, showing an increased prevalence of stress, anxiety and insecurity [31]. Female students were found to be affected more than males, with a high risk for developing depression and negative emotional states, which was associated with an increase in leisure time and decreased physical activity [30]. Therefore, examining these factors can play a key role in developing public health policies to minimize the psychological impact among future dentists.

7.2. Quality of Dental Education

The COVID-19 pandemic has considerably affected the quality of dental students' training. Dentistry is a scientific–educational field which combines theoretical concepts and principles with the acquisition of practical skills. In the absence of a mandatory residency program, basic dental education requires sufficient preclinical and clinical training to ensure an adequate level of competence for future professionals in the field [32]. While distance learning could be a commonly adopted strategy for higher education in various fields, a unique challenge for dental education is the dependence on the requirements of clinical experience to achieve minimal competency in performing dental treatments [33]. Since many dental procedures produce considerable amounts of aerosols and droplets, many routine and elective dental treatments were suspended during the pandemic, thus affecting the training of dental students [1].

7.3. Dental Research

The COVID-19 pandemic has greatly impacted research in the dental field. In some cases, having limited access to patients delayed and even compromised the results of clinical trials and restricted the implementation of new ones. For example, saliva and crevicular fluids are valuable diagnostic tools in dental medicine [34,35]. Diagnostics based on salivary matrix metalloproteinases (MMPs) that can successfully quantify periodontal inflammation should be cautiously used because of potential contamination risks [35–37]. To overcome these hazards, other methods have been employed, such as the finite element method (FEM), which uses mathematical models to simulate clinical reality and does not involve patient contact [38,39]. FEM proved to be an extremely useful and reliable alternative option during the COVID-19 pandemic by providing optimal prognoses and validating different protocols of treatment in various dental specialties, such as periodontics, orthodontics or prosthodontics [39–43].

8. Perspectives and Limitations

The COVID-19 pandemic has affected and still continues to significantly impact the delivery of dental healthcare due to changing clinical protocols and adapting them in order to minimize contamination risks. Teledentistry has expanded its initial scope and, when correctly implemented, could be an effective tool, but should be considered as a complementary means rather than an alternative to on-site, conventional treatments that are based on the principle of personalized medicine. Teledentistry can offer tremendous benefits in the delivery of some applications, while it can be limited in others. For example, pre- and post-operative counselling, education and care, nutrition advice and quick access to images of oral cavities through user-friendly imaging devices accessible to patients can all be performed via teledentistry. On the other hand, there are many challenges associated with teledentistry. These are primarily related to the lack of guidelines, standardization and scientific validation of teledentistry procedures and tools used in addition to issues related to data security and privacy. Other constraints are related to the inability to perform a clinical tactile exam, lack of direct contact with the patients, risk of misdiagnosis, lack of technological infrastructure, poor access to the Internet, lack of hardware, low information technology literacy, resistance to new technologies, and a lack of training and consumer awareness. There is no "one-fit-all" solution to overcome these challenges, and as the field evolves, new creative models will be developed in order to fit particular scenarios. Irrespective of the model used, the patient should be provided with the same quality of dental care as performed in the clinic. As a minimum, it should meet the following criteria: provide easy access to all populations, including the underserved, provide oral health delivery, including specialty care in a timely manner, and be sustainable, affordable and time effective. There are several limitations of this narrative review that include the inherent lack of quantitative analyses of published studies and being prone to biases. Notwithstanding, teledentistry proved to be useful in enhancing communication with, and treatment of, various categories of patients, such as those from nursing homes and prisons, and it is cost and time efficient. It is readily accessible, user friendly, and will no doubt continue to be expanded to new areas of dentistry and remote dental services, even after the COVID-19 pandemic. Moving forward, teledentistry will play a significant role in dental education and curriculum delivery by using technological advances in offering the skills required to maintain the quality of care while minimizing disease transmission. Finally, there is a need for more long-term comprehensive studies evaluating the impact of teledentistry in prevention, clinical outcomes and delivery of treatment across all branches of dentistry, as well as in developing distant training protocols in order to provide dental education in a safe environment.

9. Conclusions

Dental staff, academic personnel, dental students and dental researchers were severely affected by the COVID-19 pandemic, which led to a decrease in the quality of care, clinical work and practical training. Despite its limitations, teledentistry has become a critically important tool during the COVID-19 pandemic in mitigating the risks of virus contamination and transmission. Overcoming challenges in adopting teledentistry by improving patient and management tools via new technologies coupled with innovations in dental engineering and equipment to minimize aerosol-transmitted pathogens will, no doubt, find the dentistry world better prepared to withstand the negative impact of a potential future pandemic. Thus, future research should focus on improving the quality and reliability of teledentistry in order to eliminate current technological errors and further integrating it as a complementary option in dental healthcare systems worldwide.

Author Contributions: Conceptualization, I.L. and A.G.; writing—original draft preparation, A.G. and D.S.; writing—review and editing, M.T.; supervision, I.L. All authors have read and agreed to the published version of the manuscript.

Funding: This research received no external funding.

Institutional Review Board Statement: Not applicable.

Informed Consent Statement: Not applicable.

Conflicts of Interest: The authors declare no conflict of interest.

References

1. Devlin, H.; Soltani, P. COVID-19 and Dentistry. *Encyclopedia* **2021**, *1*, 496–504. [CrossRef]
2. Darvish, S.; Salman, B.N. General Considerations for the Practice of Pediatric Dentistry in the Period of COVID-19 pandemic: A Review. *J. Biosci. Med.* **2021**, *9*, 29–42. [CrossRef]
3. Senpuku, H.; Fukumoto, M.; Uchiyama, T.; Taguchi, C.; Suzuki, I.; Arikawa, K. Effects of Extraoral Suction on Droplets and Aerosols for Infection Control Practices. *Dent. J.* **2021**, *9*, 80. [CrossRef] [PubMed]
4. Xu, J.; Li, Y.; Gan, F.; Du, Y.; Yao, Y. Salivary Glands: Potential Reservoirs for COVID-19 Asymptomatic Infection. *J. Dent. Res.* **2020**, *99*, 989. [CrossRef]
5. Giraudeau, N. Teledentistry and COVID-19: Be Mindful of Bogus "Good" Ideas! *Inquiry* **2021**, *58*, 00469580211015050. [CrossRef]
6. Butera, A.; Maiorani, C.; Natoli, V.; Bruni, A.; Coscione, C.; Magliano, G.; Giacobbo, G.; Morelli, A.; Moressa, S.; Scribante, A. Bio-Inspired Systems in Nonsurgical Periodontal Therapy to Reduce Contaminated Aerosol during COVID-19: A Comprehensive and Bibliometric Review. *J. Clin. Med.* **2020**, *9*, 3914. [CrossRef]
7. Kwok, Y.L.A.; Gralton, J.; McLaws, M.L. Face Touching: A Frequent Habit that Has Implications for Hand Hygiene. *Am. J. Infect. Control* **2020**, *43*, 112–114. [CrossRef]
8. Salgarello, S.; Salvadori, M.; Mazzoleni, F.; Francinelli, J.; Bertoletti, P.; Audino, E.; Garo, M.L. The New Normalcy in Dentistry after the COVID-19 Pandemic: An Italian Cross-Sectional Survey. *Dent. J.* **2021**, *9*, 86. [CrossRef]

9. Vergara-Buenaventura, A.; Castro-Ruiz, C. Use of mouthwashes against COVID-19 in dentistry. *Br. J. Oral Maxillofac. Surg.* **2020**, *58*, 924–927. [CrossRef]
10. Kappenberg-Nitescu, D.C.; Luchian, I.; Martu, I.; Solomon, S.; Martu, S.; Pasarin, L.; Martu, A.; Sioustis, I.A.; Goriuc, A.; Tatarciuc, M. Periodontal effects of two innovative oral rinsing substances in oncologic patients. *Exp. Ther. Med.* **2021**, *21*, 1. [CrossRef]
11. Scarano, A.; Inchingolo, F.; Lorusso, F. Environmental Disinfection of a Dental Clinic during the COVID-19 Pandemic: A Narrative Insight. *BioMed Res. Int.* **2020**, *1*, 15. [CrossRef] [PubMed]
12. Meethil, A.P.; Saraswat, S.; Chaudhary, P.P.; Dabdoub, S.M.; Kumar, P.S. Sources of SARS-CoV-2 and Other Microorganisms in Dental Aerosols. *J. Dent. Res.* **2021**, *100*, 817–823. [CrossRef] [PubMed]
13. Nijakowski, K.; Cieślik, K.; Łaganowski, K.; Gruszczyński, D.; Surdacka, A. The Impact of the COVID-19 Pandemic on the Spectrum of Performed Dental Procedures. *Int. J. Environ. Res. Public Health* **2021**, *18*, 3421. [CrossRef] [PubMed]
14. Benzian, H.; Beltrán-Aguilar, E.; Niederman, R. Systemic Management of Pandemic Risks in Dental Practice: A Consolidated Framework for COVID-19 Control in Dentistry. *Front. Med.* **2021**, *8*, 196. [CrossRef]
15. Expósito-Delgado, A.J.; Ausina-Márquez, V.; Mateos-Moreno, M.V.; Martínez-Sanz, E.; del Carmen Trullols-Casas, M.; Llamas-Ortuño, M.E.; Blanco-González, J.M.; Almerich-Torres, T.; Bravo, M.; Martínez-Beneyto, Y. Delivery of Health Care by Spanish Dental Hygienists in Private and Public Dental Services during the COVID-19 De-Escalation Phase (June 2020): A Cross-Sectional Study. *Int. J. Environ. Res. Public Health* **2021**, *18*, 8298. [CrossRef]
16. Ghai, S. Teledentistry during COVID-19 pandemic. *Diabetes Metab. Syndr.* **2020**, *14*, 933–935. [CrossRef]
17. Giudice, A.; Barone, S.; Muraca, D.; Averta, F.; Diodati, F.; Antonelli, A.; Fortunato, L. Can Teledentistry Improve the Monitoring of Patients during the COVID-19 Dissemination? A Descriptive Pilot Study. *Int. J. Environ. Res. Public Health.* **2020**, *17*, 3399. [CrossRef]
18. Dusseja, S.H.; Dinesh, R.; Panwar, S.; Safna, A. Patients' Views Regarding Dental Concerns and Tele dentistry during COVID-19 Pandemic. *Int. J. Environ. Res. Public Health.* **2020**, *5*, 423–429.
19. Machado, R.A.; Souza, N.L.; Oliveira, R.M.; Martelli Junior, H.; Bonan, P.R.F. Social media and telemedicine for oral diagnosis and counselling in the COVID-19 era. *Oral Oncol.* **2020**, *105*, 104685. [CrossRef]
20. Estai, M.; Kruger, E.; Tennant, M.; Bunt, S.; Kanagasingam, Y. Challenges in the uptake of telemedicine in dentistry. *Rural Remote Health* **2016**, *16*, 3915. [CrossRef]
21. Kappenberg-Niţescu, D.C.; Păsărin, L.; Mârţu, S.; Teodorescu, C.; Vasiliu, B.; Mârţu, I.; Luchian, I.; Solomon, S.M. Determining Chemotherapy Agents in Saliva through Spectrometry and Chromatography Methods Correlated with Periodontal Status in Oncology Patients. *Appl. Sci.* **2021**, *11*, 5984. [CrossRef]
22. Madi, M.; Kumar, M.; Pentapati, K.C.; Vineetha, R. Smart-phone based telemedicine: Instant messaging application as a platform for radiographic interpretations of jaw pathologies. *J. Oral Biol. Craniofac. Res.* **2021**, *11*, 368–372. [CrossRef] [PubMed]
23. Torul, D.; Kahveci, K.; Kahveci, C. Is Tele-Dentistry an Effective Approach for Patient Follow-up in Maxillofacial Surgery. *J. Maxillofac. Oral Surg.* **2021**, *20*, 1–7. [CrossRef] [PubMed]
24. Wallace, C.K.; Schofield, C.E.; Burbridge, L.A.L.; O'Donnell, K.L. Role of teledentistry in paediatric dentistry. *Br. Dent. J.* **2021**, 1–6. [CrossRef] [PubMed]
25. Mekhemar, M.; Attia, S.; Dörfer, C.; Conrad, J. Dental Nurses' Mental Health in Germany: A Nationwide Survey during the COVID-19 Pandemic. *Int. J. Environ. Res. Public Health* **2021**, *18*, 8108. [CrossRef]
26. Schmidt, J.; Perina, V.; Treglerova, J.; Pilbauerova, N.; Suchanek, J.; Smucler, R. COVID-19 Prevalence among Czech Dentists. *Int. J. Environ. Res. Public Health* **2021**, *18*, 12488. [CrossRef] [PubMed]
27. Koç, Y.; Akyüz, S.; Akşit-Bıçak, D. Clinical Experience, Knowledge, Attitudes and Practice of Turkish Pediatric Dentists during the COVID-19 Pandemic. *Medicina* **2021**, *57*, 1140. [CrossRef]
28. Morgado, M.; Mendes, J.J.; Proença, L. COVID-19 Risk Perception and Confidence among Clinical Dental Students: Impact on Patient Management. *Med. Sci. Forum* **2021**, *5*, 26. [CrossRef]
29. Balkaran, R.; Bhat, M.; Smith, W.; Marchan, S. COVID-19 Stressors among Dental Academics at UWI—A Caribbean Perspective. *Oral* **2021**, *1*, 5. [CrossRef]
30. Mekhemar, M.; Attia, S.; Dörfer, C.; Conrad, J. Dental Students in Germany throughout the COVID-19 Pandemic: A Psychological Assessment and Cross-Sectional Survey. *Biology* **2021**, *10*, 611. [CrossRef]
31. Zarzecka, J.; Zarzecka-Francica, E.; Gala, A.; Gębczyński, K.; Pihut, M. Dental environmental stress during the COVID-19 pandemic at the Jagiellonian University Medical College, Kraków, Poland. *Int. J. Occup. Med. Environ. Health* **2021**, *34*, 211–222. [CrossRef] [PubMed]
32. Hassan, M.G.; Amer, H. Dental Education in the Time of COVID-19 Pandemic: Challenges and Recommendations. *Front. Med.* **2021**, *8*, 648899. [CrossRef] [PubMed]
33. Talapko, J.; Perić, I.; Vulić, P.; Pustijanac, E.; Jukić, M.; Bekić, S.; Meštrović, T.; Škrlec, I. Mental Health and Physical Activity in Health-Related University Students during the COVID-19 Pandemic. *Healthcare* **2021**, *9*, 801. [CrossRef] [PubMed]
34. Teodorescu, A.C.; Martu, I.; Teslaru, S.; Kappenberg-Nitescu, D.C.; Goriuc, A.; Luchian, I.; Martu, M.A.; Solomon, S.M.; Martu, S. Assessment of Salivary Levels of RANKL and OPG in Aggressive versus Chronic Periodontitis. *J. Immunol. Res.* **2019**, *2019*, 6195258. [CrossRef] [PubMed]
35. Luchian, I.; Moscalu, M.; Goriuc, A.; Nucci, L.; Tatarciuc, M.; Martu, I.; Covasa, M. Using Salivary MMP-9 to Successfully Quantify Periodontal Inflammation during Orthodontic Treatment. *J. Clin. Med.* **2021**, *10*, 379. [CrossRef] [PubMed]

36. Wang, W.K.; Chen, S.Y.; Liu, I.J.; Chen, Y.C.; Chen, H.L.; Yang, C.F.; Chen, P.J.; Yeh, S.H.; Kao, C.L.; Huang, L.M.; et al. Detection of SARS-Associated Coronavirus in Throat Wash and Saliva in Early Diagnosis. *Emerg. Infect. Dis.* **2004**, *10*, 1213–1219. [CrossRef] [PubMed]
37. Sabino-Silva, R.; Jardim, A.C.G.; Siqueira, W.L. Coronavirus COVID-19 Impacts to Dentistry and Potential Salivary Diagnosis. *Clin. Oral Investig.* **2020**, *24*, 1619–1621. [CrossRef]
38. Luchian, I.; Vata, I.; Martu, I.; Stirbu, C.; Tatarciuc, M.; Martu, S. The periodontal effects of an optimal intrusive force on a maxillary central incisor. A FEM evaluation. *Rom. J. Oral Rehab.* **2016**, *8*, 51–55.
39. Luchian, I.; Martu, M.-A.; Tatarciuc, M.; Scutariu, M.M.; Ioanid, N.; Pasarin, L.; Kappenberg-Nitescu, D.C.; Sioustis, I.-A.; Solomon, S.M. Using FEM to Assess the Effect of Orthodontic Forces on Affected Periodontium. *Appl. Sci.* **2021**, *11*, 7183. [CrossRef]
40. Tatarciuc, M.; Maftei, G.A.; Vitalariu, A.; Luchian, I.; Martu, I.; Diaconu-Popa, D. Inlay-Retained Dental Bridges—A Finite Element Analysis. *Appl. Sci.* **2021**, *11*, 3770. [CrossRef]
41. Sioustis, I.-A.; Axinte, M.; Prelipceanu, M.; Martu, A.; Kappenberg-Nitescu, D.-C.; Teslaru, S.; Luchian, I.; Solomon, S.M.; Cimpoesu, N.; Martu, S. Finite Element Analysis of Mandibular Anterior Teeth with Healthy, but Reduced Periodontium. *Appl. Sci.* **2021**, *11*, 3824. [CrossRef]
42. Devlin, A. Post-pandemic dentistry—Restart or reform? *Br. Dent. J.* **2021**, *230*, 306. [CrossRef] [PubMed]
43. Martu, M.A.; Maftei, G.A.; Sufaru, I.G.; Jelihovschi, I.; Luchian, I.; Hurjui, L.; Martu, I.; Pasarin, L. COVID-19 and Periodontal Disease-Ethiopathogenic and Clinical Implications. *Rom. J. Oral Rehab.* **2020**, *12*, 116–124.

MDPI
St. Alban-Anlage 66
4052 Basel
Switzerland
www.mdpi.com

International Journal of Environmental Research and Public Health Editorial Office
E-mail: ijerph@mdpi.com
www.mdpi.com/journal/ijerph

www.ingramcontent.com/pod-product-compliance
Lightning Source LLC
LaVergne TN
LVHW070608100526
838202LV00012B/597